NON-ALCOHOLIC FATTY LIVER DISEASE - MOLECULAR BASES, PREVENTION AND TREATMENT

Edited by **Rodrigo Valenzuela**

Non-Alcoholic Fatty Liver Disease - Molecular Bases, Prevention and Treatment

http://dx.doi.org/10.5772/68045
Edited by Rodrigo Valenzuela

Contributors

Kaori Minehira, Monjur Ahmed, Levent Doganay, Seyma Katrinli, Kamil Ozdil, Gizem Dinler-Doganay, Kingsley Pereko, Jacob Setorglo, Joyce Tiweh, Matilda Steiner-Asiedu, Shahinul Alam, Thupten Kelsang Lama., Golam Mustafa, Mahabubul Alam, Nooruddin Ahmad, Monica Lupsor-Platon, Parkash, Subha Saeed, Ian Martins

Published by InTech
Janeza Trdine 9, 51000 Rijeka, Croatia

Notice

Statements and opinions expressed in the chapters are these of the individual contributors and not necessarily those of the editors or publisher. No responsibility is accepted for the accuracy of information contained in the published chapters. The publisher assumes no responsibility for any damage or injury to persons or property arising out of the use of any materials, instructions, methods or ideas contained in the book.

Publishing Process Manager Romina Skomersic
Technical Editor SPi Global
Cover InTech Design team

First published March, 2018
Printed in Croatia
Legal deposit, Croatia: National and University Library in Zagreb

Additional hard copies can be obtained from orders@intechopen.com

Non-Alcoholic Fatty Liver Disease - Molecular Bases, Prevention and Treatment, Edited by Rodrigo Valenzuela
p. cm.
Print ISBN 978-953-51-3923-2
Online ISBN 978-953-51-3924-9

For EU product safety concerns:
IN TECH d.o.o., Prolaz Marije Krucifikse Kozulić 3, 51000 Rijeka, Croatia,
info@intechopen.com or visit our website at intechopen.com.

Meet the editor

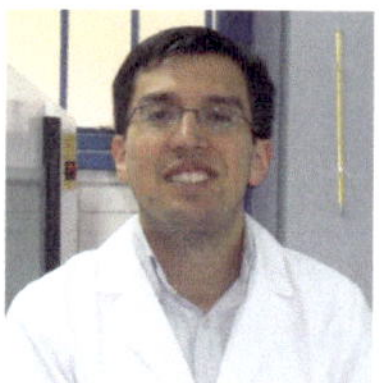

Rodrigo Valenzuela completed his pre-graduate studies (Nutritionist) (2003), master's degree in Nutrition and Food Science (2007), and doctoral degree in Nutrition and Food at the University of Chile (2012). Currently, he is a research scientist in Nutrition and Food Science and an assistant professor in Nutrition and Food, in Health and Disease Section, and in the Nutrition Department, Faculty of Medicine, University of Chile. His current research areas are in lipids in health and disease, metabolism and hepato-protective effects of polyunsaturated fatty acid from marine and vegetable origin, liver steatosis prevention by dietary interventions in animal models, and physiological effects of different bioactive compounds as functional food. He wrote sixty research publications, related with the food and nutrition in health and disease.

Contents

Preface

Non-alcoholic fatty liver disease (NAFLD) is characterized by an excessive and pathological accumulation of fat in hepatocytes (> 5% of the total weight of the liver). It is characterized by (i) the presence of hepatic steatosis as determined by imaging or histological diagnosis and (ii) the absence of secondary cause for accumulation of fat, such as excessive alcohol consumption (> 20 g/day in men and 10 g/day in women). In addition, with NAFLD, it is possible to identify a wide spectrum of pathologies including simple steatosis (fat infiltration), steatohepatitis (involving inflammation), and cirrhosis, with a worldwide prevalence of 10 to 46%. In this context, NAFLD is considered the hepatic manifestation of the metabolic syndrome, and among its risk factors, obesity, diabetes mellitus type 2 (DM2), insulin resistance, and dyslipidemia are noteworthy. On the other hand, polymorphisms in lipid metabolism genes, cytokine regulation, fibrotic mediators, and oxidative stress have shown a possible association with the onset and progression of NAFLD. Lifestyles such as physical inactivity and unhealthy diet are risk factors for obesity and cardiometabolic disorders, leading to the development of metabolic syndrome and NAFLD, through the development of insulin resistance, oxidative stress, and inflammation.

The metabolism of nutrients are altered in subjects with NAFLD, with an increase in the production of reactive oxygen species, generating oxidative stress, mitochondrial dysfunction, reticulum stress, and a pro-inflammatory and pro-lipogenic state at the liver level. For this reason, with the development of NAFLD, diet plays a fundamental role; the Western diet is characterized by a high intake of energy from cereal, simple carbohydrates (sugar), fats (mainly saturated and trans-fatty acids), and high-fructose corn syrup (especially in sugary drinks), as well as a low consumption of fruits, vegetables, and fish rich in n-3 fatty acids, exacerbating the hepatic fat accumulation.

NAFLD is associated with the main factors of metabolic syndrome, such as obesity, characterized by dysfunctional visceral adiposity and a chronic inflammatory state that induces insulin resistance. In this regard, the insulin resistance observed in both the liver and peripheral tissues favors an increase in lipolysis. This high mobilization of lipids, specifically free fatty acids from adipose tissue to the liver, increases hepatic lipogenesis and exacerbates the deposition of triglycerides in hepatocytes, which leads to an increase in mitochondrial activity and production of oxygen reactive species and oxidative stress. In this context, the theory of the "two strokes" of Day and James tries to explain the pathogenesis and progression of NAFLD. The "first stroke" is the reversible hepatic accumulation of triglycerides, due to insulin resistance, resulting in metabolic and molecular alterations, increasing the susceptibility to the "second stroke" represented by the oxidative stress that causes inflammation and tissue injury. In recent years, the theory of "multiple parallel blows" has emerged, where the insulin resistance is the "central blow," making the hepatocyte susceptible to (i) production of oxygen reactive species by oxidation of free fatty acids, (ii) dysregulation in the production of cytokines, and (iii) mitochondrial dysfunction, leading to the appearance and progression of NAFLD.

Collectively, this book intends to present a systematic and comprehensive review of NAFLD, highlighting its epidemiological and molecular aspects, as well as its prevention and treatment.

Rodrigo Valenzuela, MSc, PhD
Nutritionist
Assistant Professor
Nutrition Department
Faculty of Medicine
University of Chile
Santiago, Chile

Section 1

General Aspect and Molecular Bases

Chapter 1

Non-alcoholic Fatty Liver Disease: What We Learn from Omics Studies

Seyma Katrinli, Kamil Ozdil,
Gizem Dinler-Doganay and Levent Doganay

Additional information is available at the end of the chapter

http://dx.doi.org/10.5772/intechopen.71025

Abstract

Non-alcoholic fatty liver disease (NAFLD) is one of the most common causes of chronic liver diseases with 10–30% prevalence in western countries. The severity of NAFLD ranges from simple steatosis to non-alcoholic steatohepatitis (NASH), cirrhosis, and hepatocellular carcinoma (HCC). However, the wide range of clinical staging of the disease prevents the clear understanding of its pathogenesis. Recently, high-throughput genomic, transcriptomic, and proteomic studies focus on enlightening the complex mechanisms responsible for NAFLD and NASH development. All together these Omics studies, in different cohorts once again, proved that NAFLD and NASH are linked with many complex mechanisms such as accumulation and traffic of various lipids in the liver and activation of inflammation responses. Moreover, some of these studies may have identified potential biomarkers and candidate risky or protective alleles that can be a valuable tool for the assessment of susceptibility and histological severity of NAFLD. Nonetheless, confirmation of these potential biomarkers and candidate genes by multiple Omics tools is required for their clinical application in the diagnosis and treatment of NASH and NAFLD.

Keywords: non-alcoholic fatty liver disease, non-alcoholic steatohepatitis, liver, genomics, proteomics, Omics, GWAS, NASH, NAFLD

1. Introduction

Non-alcoholic fatty liver disease (NAFLD) is a serious hepatic disorder, affecting up to 30% of the general population of Western countries and approximately 15% in Asian population [1, 2]. The increased prevalence in developing countries is related with sedentary life style and lack of exercise. Moreover, the increase in NAFLD prevalence is also related with alterations in dietary intake caused by urban lifestyle which is represented by a 24% augmented energy intake because of the enhancements in the consumption of flour, cereal products, and added sugar and fats and/or in total fat and fruit intake [3]. In addition, the use of corn syrup or high fructose as sweeteners in beverages greatly contributed the prevalence of NAFLD [4]. Hence, various dietary models are being evaluated for prevention of NAFLD. The top studied dietary interventions include diets restricted in calories and carbohydrates with soy protein addition, low calorie diet rich in proteins, high protein diet, soft drinks with fructose compared to glucose sodas, and Mediterranean diet [5]. The fact that NAFLD is the second most common reason for liver transplantation emphasizes the burden of NAFLD to public health [6]. NAFLD comprises an entire pathological spectrum of diseases with successive stages of increasing severity, ranging from simple steatosis (SS), non-alcoholic steatohepatitis (NASH), and cirrhosis to hepatocellular carcinoma (HCC) [7]. The end result, HCC, is the fifth common cancer among all primary neoplastic diseases and affects one million individuals annually worldwide. Despite the common fact that hepatitis B or hepatitis C infection-associated liver cirrhosis or abusive alcohol consumption is the primary cause of HCC, recent studies reported that HCCs may also affect non-cirrhotic livers, most of them having no associated risk factors. Consequently, NASH is now evaluated as a significant risk factor due to the high prevalence of obesity and type 2 diabetes mellitus [8]. Recent reports stated that the risk to develop HCC in patients with metabolic syndrome is increased by 2.13 (odd ratio), while the increase rate is 4.4 in patients with NAFLD [9, 10].

NAFLD is closely associated with obesity, combined hyperlipidemia, type II diabetes mellitus, high blood pressure, and insulin resistance; it can be regarded as the hepatic manifestation of metabolic syndrome [11]. Insulin resistance, dyslipidemia, and cardiovascular risk factors are known to arise from abnormalities in fatty acid metabolism and systemic inflammation, but the exact link between metabolic syndrome and the onset and progression of liver injury is still unclear [12]. Steatosis, characterized by an accumulation of triglycerides in the liver parenchyma, may develop into NAFLD if the rates of hepatic uptake of circulating blood free fatty acids (FFA), which originates from excessive adipose tissue lipolysis, and de novo liver lipogenesis from glucose are greater than the rate of mitochondrial fatty acid oxidation or export as triglycerides within low-density lipoproteins. This phenomenon arises from abnormalities in glucose, fatty acid, and lipoprotein metabolism accompanied by the development of insulin resistance. On the other hand, upcoming evidence now suggest that triglyceride accumulation in the form of lipid droplets could instead be a parameter of excessive fatty acid trafficking, while non-triglyceride fatty acid metabolites would be the consequence of lipotoxicity of the NASH pathogenesis [13]. Insulin resistance results in an excessive flow of fatty acids from the adipose tissue and also hinders peripheral glucose removal. In the liver, fatty acid disposal causes excessive production of reactive oxygen species, followed by lipid peroxidation and augmented inflammatory response [14]. Still, the exact mechanism that explains progression of SS to NASH is not yet fully clear. Currently, liver biopsy is still the gold standard in diagnosis of NAFLD. The histological indication of NAFLD is determined as lipid accumulation in the hepatocytes in the absence of pathologies such as viral hepatitis or alcohol abuse [15]. However, liver biopsy has certain disadvantages. First and most important of all, it is an invasive procedure. Moreover, since NAFLD does not uniformly affect liver, this heterogeneity may cause some biases in biopsy results [16, 17]. Hence, there is an urgent need for non-invasive biomarkers to assess liver diseases such as NAFLD.

Currently, high-throughput Omics studies engage in to solve the complex mechanisms responsible for NAFLD and NASH development. The genomic studies focus on genome-wide association studies (GWAS) that identify biomarkers across whole genomes to determine genetic variations associated with a disease of interest. The technologies of high-throughput genotyping are now able to assay the common single nucleotide polymorphism (SNP) and find the association between SNPs and clinical conditions or measurable traits [18]. As in many other diseases, besides genetic factors epigenetics and transcriptomic alterations are involved in the development of NAFLD and NASH. Additionally, identification of specific proteins, either as novel biomarkers or as over-/under-expressed markers through proteomic studies, may have a massive effect by increasing the availability of biomarkers for early diagnosis and therapy [19].

The development of NAFLD is a complex multifactorial process that involves the disruption of multiple gene and protein mechanisms. Initially, Day and James suggested a "two-hit hypothesis" to define the development of NAFLD: The "first hit" corresponds to a primary hepatic lipid accumulation which is described as steatosis; the "second hit" is an oxidative stress leading to lipid peroxidation, followed by liver injury and inflammation [20]. Recently, this traditional "two-hit hypothesis" has been upgraded to "multiple parallel hits hypothesis." It has been proposed that significant overlaps among insulin resistance, hepatic de novo lipogenesis, and subsequent hepatocyte injury also come into play in the progression from SS to NASH [21]. In addition, various candidate gene studies focusing on genetic factors of NAFLD development have further supported the "multiple parallel hits hypothesis" [22]. This review aims to sum up the current Omics studies such as genomics, transcriptomics, and proteomics to offer a better understanding of the pathogenesis of NAFLD.

2. Genomics in NAFLD

Accomplishment of Human Genome Project in 2003 greatly accelerates genome-wide association studies (GWAS) that enable researchers to identify biomarkers across genomes of population that are associated with a given disease. GWAS has a unique hypothesis-free approach that comes handy for examining genes that otherwise would have not been considered as candidates because of our limited knowledge of their function and for revealing as well non-protein coding regions of the genome that involve crucial regulatory alterations [14]. Thus, there are multiple GWAS conducted to identify genes that are associated with the development of NAFLD. According to genomic studies, the associated genes with the pathophysiology of NAFLD belong to hepatic lipid metabolism, ECM balance, cytokines, and insulin resistance [11] (**Table 1**).

The first GWA study that was performed by Romeo et al. notably increased the notion that genetic factors could affect the susceptibility of NAFLD [24]. In their study, Romeo et al. presented the association between a genome-wide survey of 9229 non-synonymous SNPs and hepatic fat detected by MR spectroscopy in 1032 African-American, 696 European-American, and 383 Hispanic adults residing in Dallas County and found that an allele in human patatin-like phospholipase domain containing 3 gene (PNPLA3) (rs738409, I148M)

Candidate genes	Cohort (n = Population size)	Reference
GGT1 and ABO	n = 7715; replication in 4704	[23]
PNPLA3	n = 11,340	[24–26]
FDFT1 and COL13A1	n = 236	[27]
PNPLA3, NCAN, PPP1R3B, CCKR, and LYPLAL1	n = 7126; replication in 592 cases and 1405 control	[28]
PNPLA3, TRIB1, CPN1, loci near HSD17B13, and MAPK10	61,089	[29]
PNPLA3 and TM6SF2	2736	[30]

GGT1, gamma-glutamyltransferase 1; PNPLA3, patatin-like phospholipase domain containing 3; FDFT1, farnesyl-diphosphate farnesyltransferase 1; COL13A1, collagen type XIII alpha 1 chain; NCAN, neurocan; PPP1R3B, protein phosphatase 1 regulatory subunit 3B; CCKR, cholecystokinin receptor; LYPLAL1, lysophospholipase-like 1; TRIB1, tribbles pseudokinase 1; CPN1, carboxypeptidase N subunit 1; HSD17B13, hydroxysteroid 17-beta dehydrogenase 13; MAPK10, mitogen-activated protein kinase 10; TM6SF2, transmembrane 6 superfamily member 2.

Table 1. GWA studies of NAFLD.

was strongly contributing increased hepatic lipid levels, alanine aminotransferase levels, and hepatic inflammation. PNPLA3 gene that encodes adiponutrin is known to have lipase activity in vitro and has been shown to be involved in glucose and lipid metabolism [24]. Recent reports also supported the importance of this variant in NASH progression owing to its connection with fibrosis development [25]. The association of this variant in PNPLA3 gene (rs738409; I148M) with the susceptibility and histological severity of NAFLD was also confirmed by the study of Sookoian and Pirola which included 2937 subjects [26]. Chalasani et al. have examined 324,623 SNPs from the 22 autosomal chromosomes in 236 non-Hispanic white women with well-diagnosed NAFLD for their clinical and histological features [27]. They reported association of SNP rs2645424 on chromosome 8 in farnesyl diphosphate farnesyl transferase 1 (FDFT1) with NAFLD activity score and SNP rs1227756 on chromosome 10 in a collagen XIII variant (COL13A1), with lobular inflammation. While they stated association of several variants with the degree of fibrosis or serum levels of alanine aminotransferase, they found no significant association between genotypes and steatosis, ballooning degeneration, portal inflammation, or other features of NAFLD. Transmembrane 6 Superfamily Member 2 (TM6SF2) gene is also found to be associated with NAFLD [30]. Minor allele frequency for the rs58542926 TM6SF2 polymorphism has been reported as 7% in Europeans, 4% in Hispanics, and 2% in African Americans [31], which are much lesser than MAF for PNPLA3 rs738409 (I148M) variant which has been reported as 49% in Hispanics, 23% in those of European ancestry, and 17% in African Americans [32]. Individuals with rs58542926 TM6SF2 polymorphism have shown to possess a greater risk of developing NAFLD (OR 2.13 (95% CI: 1.36–3.30)) [33]. Another GWAS conducted by Yuan et al. in three populations (total n = 7715) with replication in three additional cohorts (total n = 4704) analyzed genetic variations affecting plasma liver enzyme levels and reported six loci that have an effect on plasma levels of liver enzymes as well as confirming previously stated associations between the GGT1 locus and gamma glutamyl transpeptidase (GGT) levels and between the ABO locus and alkaline phosphatase levels [23].

Altogether, this numerous genomic studies propose the association of several genetic factors, especially those responsible for lipid metabolism, with NAFLD development. Still, further studies are required to deeply understand the effect of genetic variations on the pathogenesis of NAFLD to develop specific therapies that prevent the progression of the disease or specific treatments at each progressive step of the disease.

3. Transcriptomics in NALFD

The development of transcriptomic tools, predominantly real-time quantitative reverse transcription polymerase chain reaction (qRT-PCR) and microarrays, accompanied by supporting informatics and statistical methodologies enables researchers to investigate alterations in global mRNA levels in NAFLD. As in many other diseases, besides genetic factors, epigenetic and transcriptomic changes participate the progression of NAFLD. The term epigenetics is described as heritable alterations in gene expression patterns that are not encoded directly within DNA but are instead determined by related factors such as DNA methylation or histone modifications. While these epigenetic changes are heritable, they can also be modified in response to environmental effects [34]. The liver, being the key metabolic organ, is subjected to nutrition-derived factors that can alter its epigenetic signature. Two essential factors that play a role in epigenetic modifications of histones and DNA are acetyl-CoA and S-adenosylmethionine which are also directly involved in glucose or methionine metabolism, respectively [35]. Consequently, histone acetylation has been shown to participate to NAFLD development by triggering lipogenic and glycolytic genes, while abnormalities in S-adenosylmethionine levels have been demonstrated to result in lipogenesis, accumulation of hepatic triglycerides, and NAFLD [35]. In terms of ease in clinical applications, it is better for an epigenetic biomarker to be discovered in peripheral blood [36]. Hereof, a promising study that examined body mass index loss in obese adolescents reported significance of altered DNA methylation in Aquaporin-9 (AQP9), dual specificity protein phosphatase 22 (DUSP22), homeodomain-interacting protein kinase 3 (HIPK3), troponin T1 (TNNT1), and troponin I3 (TNNI3) genes [37].

MicroRNAs (miRNAs) which are short RNA molecules of about 22 nucleotides that control mRNA stability and thus transcription levels are crucial transcriptomic factors that can affect NAFLD development [14]. Studies have inconsistent results for their involvement in steatosis, possibly due to the variances of diagnostic methods, staging, and miRNA measurement [38]. The direct analysis of miRNA in the blood makes them ideal biomarkers for the distinct stages of steatosis. Recently, specific microarrays, such as muParaflo microRNA microarrays, greatly contributed to the examination of microRNAs in NAFLD. For instance, the expression miRNA-122, which constitutes 70% of the total liver miRNAs, has been shown to be augmented in the blood of NAFLD patients [39, 40]. The study of Cermelli et al. that compares miRNA levels of NALFD patients and healthy controls reported increased miRNA-34a and miRNA-16 levels in NAFLD patients. Also, they suggested that miRNA-122 and miRNA-34a might be a useful biomarker for the evaluation of NAFLD and NASH [39]. Besides miRNA-122, Pirola et al. reported association of miRNA-192 and miRNA-375 with the severity of the disease [40]. Nonetheless, since there is a dynamic and multifactorial relationship between miRNAs and gene regulation, further studies and careful evaluations are required before miRNAs can be used as biomarkers in the diagnosis and staging of NAFLD.

In addition to epigenetic factors and miRNAs, alterations in gene expression profile also affect progression to NAFLD. Several cross-sectional studies performed on cohorts with various histological parameters (alcoholic steatohepatitis and NASH vs. no NASH, NASH vs. no NASH, control vs. steatosis vs. NASH, control vs. steatosis vs. NASH with steatosis >5% vs. NASH with steatosis <5%) reported the significant effect of Wnt pathway as a protagonist, besides genes participated in absorption, distribution, metabolism, and excretion (ADME); aldose reductase AKR1B10; and keratin family member KRT23 [41–45]. Studies also revealed that genes involved in cellular proliferation and ECM organization, such as dermatopontin (DPT), were differentially expressed in the liver transcriptome of NAFLD patients [46–48]. Unfortunately, subtle alterations in individual's gene expression caused by interindividual heterogeneity of the disease and the adaptive nature of the pathological response limit clear-cut identification of patient categories and therefore complicate identification of transcriptomic biomarkers [41, 43, 45, 48].

4. Proteomics in NAFLD

The improvement of novel proteomic tools accelerated researches in NAFLD diagnosis and discovery of biomarkers. The first study that examined serum protein profiles in NAFLD by surface-enhanced laser desorption ionization time of flight mass spectrometry (SELDI-TOF MS) on 98 obese patients, with 91 NAFLD patients (12 steatosis alone, 52 steatosis with non-specific inflammation, 27 NASH) and 7 patients without NAFLD as obese control, reported 12 significant protein peaks. However, because of the inherent limitation of low mass accuracy in SELDI-TOF MS, researchers could only identify fibrinogen γ and proposed a possible association with fibrosis [49]. The study of Bell et al. identified significant alterations in 55 proteins between NAFLD and NASH with advanced fibrosis by performing an ion-intensity-based, label-free quantitative proteomic approach (LFQP) [50]. They also reported significant changes of 15 proteins between early NASH and NASH with progressed fibrosis. From their data, a 6-protein diagnostic method that includes fibrinogen β chain, retinol-binding protein 4, serum amyloid P component, lumican, transgelin 2, and CD5 antigen-like and a 3-protein diagnostic method consisting of component C7, insulin-like growth factor acid labile subunit, and transgelin 2 were developed to diagnose the progressive stages of NAFLD (AUROC ranging from 0.83 to 0.91). Moreover, they also presented that alanine aminotransferase (ALT) was a low-grade diagnostic protein for the evaluation of different stages of NAFLD (AUROC = 0.53) [50]. Several other studies were also consistent with the fact that ALT is not a suitable NAFLD diagnosis biomarker, and no optimal ALT levels are present to evaluate advanced fibrosis [51]. Even with the inability to discover unique biomarkers that could distinguish between NAFLD and NASH, the study of Bell et al. greatly contributed into the understanding of the pathogenesis of NAFLD and NASH [50]. Generally, most of the proteins identified by several proteomic studies suggest

Protein categories	Protein markers	Reference
Protein carrier	Apolipoproteins	[52]
	CD5 molecule-like (CD5L)	[53]
Metabolic pathways	Carbamoyl phosphate synthetase I (CPS1)	[54]
	Glucose-regulated protein 78 (GRP78)	[54]
	Uric acid	[55]
Acute phase protein	High sensitive C-reactive protein (Hs-CRP)	[56]
	Hemoglobin	[57]
	Serum fucosylated haptoglobin (Fuc-Hpt)	[58]
	Pentraxin 3 (PTX-3)	[59]
Anti-inflammatory and antioxidant	Bilirubin	[60]
Extracellular matrix	Hyaluronic acid	[61]
	Type IV collagen 7S	[62]
	Laminin	[63]
	Lumican	[64]
	Matrix metallopeptidase 9 (MMP-9)	[65, 66]
Immune cells and cytokines	C—C motif chemokine ligand 2 (CCL2) and Monocyte chemotactic protein 1(MCP1)	[67]
	Retinol-binding protein 4 (RBP4)	[50, 68–70]

Table 2. Proteomic studies of NAFLD.

the association of immune system regulation, inflammation, hepatic ECM structure, and protein carriers in the blood with NAFLD (**Table 2**). Nonetheless, even proteomics is a great tool for gaining deep insight on the pathogenesis and progression of the disease; unfortunately, these tools cannot yet offer specific biomarkers with major clinical value to diagnose NASH or discriminate NASH and steatosis.

5. Conclusions

In conclusion, the Omics studies explained throughout the review supported the fact that NAFLD is a complex disease caused by several phenomena such as accumulation and traffic of various lipids in the liver and triggered inflammation responses. Altogether genomic, transcriptomic, and proteomic studies are in accordance with the basic detectable pathogenic mechanisms of NAFLD which are mitochondrial energetic and structural abnormalities, triggered inflammatory response via multiple targets, and lipotoxicity.

Advances in genomic and transcriptomic tools allow researchers to inspect significant genetic polymorphisms and epigenetic alterations, along with miRNA levels in different stages of the NAFLD progression. Noticeably, individuals with unfavorable genetic polymorphisms coupled with disadvantageous biological environment carry a high risk of developing NAFLD. Moreover, development of novel proteomic methodologies also supported the biomarker studies in NAFLD which aim to discover key protein molecules that carry significant clinical importance in the concourse of the disease. Even though a few candidate serum protein markers achieve to distinguish NAFLD and NASH, further validation studies of these biomarkers in larger cohorts are still required before they can be clinically used in the diagnosis and evaluation of the disease progression. Overall, further advancement of Omics studies is still required to deeply understand the pathophysiology of NAFLD and discover specific biomarkers for clinical use.

Author details

Seyma Katrinli[1,2], Kamil Ozdil[3], Gizem Dinler-Doganay[2] and Levent Doganay[3*]

*Address all correspondence to: ldoganay@hotmail.com

1 Department of Molecular Biology and Genetics, Istinye University, Istanbul, Turkey

2 Department of Molecular Biology and Genetics, Istanbul Technical University, Istanbul, Turkey

3 Department of Gastroenterology, Umraniye Teaching and Research Hospital, University of Health Sciences, Istanbul, Turkey

References

[1] Vernon G, Baranova A, Younossi ZM. Systematic review: The epidemiology and natural history of non-alcoholic fatty liver disease and non-alcoholic steatohepatitis in adults. Alimentary Pharmacology & Therapeutics. 2011;**34**(3):274-285

[2] de Alwis NM, Day CP. Non-alcoholic fatty liver disease: The mist gradually clears. Journal of Hepatology. 2008;**48**(Suppl 1):S104-S112

[3] Tappy L, Le KA, Tran C, Paquot N. Fructose and metabolic diseases: New findings, new questions. Nutrition. 2010;**26**(11-12):1044-1049

[4] Abid A, Taha O, Nseir W, Farah R, Grosovski M, Assy N. Soft drink consumption is associated with fatty liver disease independent of metabolic syndrome. Journal of Hepatology. 2009;**51**(5):918-924

[5] Hernandez-Rodas MC, Valenzuela R, Videla LA. Relevant aspects of nutritional and dietary interventions in non-alcoholic fatty liver disease. International Journal of Molecular Sciences. 2015;**16**(10):25168-25198

[6] Baffy G, Brunt EM, Caldwell SH. Hepatocellular carcinoma in non-alcoholic fatty liver disease: An emerging menace. Journal of Hepatology. 2012;**56**(6):1384-1391

[7] Qureshi K, Abrams GA. Metabolic liver disease of obesity and role of adipose tissue in the pathogenesis of nonalcoholic fatty liver disease. World Journal of Gastroenterology. 2007;**13**(26):3540-3553

[8] Yasui K, Hashimoto E, Komorizono Y, Koike K, Arii S, Imai Y, et al. Characteristics of patients with nonalcoholic steatohepatitis who develop hepatocellular carcinoma. Clinical Gastroenterology and Hepatology. 2011;**9**(5):428-433 quiz e50

[9] Welzel TM, Graubard BI, Zeuzem S, El-Serag HB, Davila JA, McGlynn KA. Metabolic syndrome increases the risk of primary liver cancer in the United States: A study in the SEER-Medicare database. Hepatology. 2011;**54**(2):463-471

[10] Sorensen HT, Mellemkjaer L, Jepsen P, Thulstrup AM, Baron J, Olsen JH, et al. Risk of cancer in patients hospitalized with fatty liver: A Danish cohort study. Journal of Clinical Gastroenterology. 2003;**36**(4):356-359

[11] Lim JW, Dillon J, Miller M. Proteomic and genomic studies of non-alcoholic fatty liver disease—Clues in the pathogenesis. World Journal of Gastroenterology. 2014;**20**(26):8325-8340

[12] Anderson N, Borlak J. Molecular mechanisms and therapeutic targets in steatosis and steatohepatitis. Pharmacological Reviews. 2008;**60**(3):311-357

[13] Neuschwander-Tetri BA. Hepatic lipotoxicity and the pathogenesis of nonalcoholic steatohepatitis: The central role of nontriglyceride fatty acid metabolites. Hepatology. 2010;**52**(2):774-788

[14] Martel C, Esposti DD, Bouchet A, Brenner C, Lemoine A. Non-alcoholic steatohepatitis: New insights from OMICS studies. Current Pharmaceutical Biotechnology. 2012;**13**(5):726-735

[15] Utzschneider KM, Review KSE. The role of insulin resistance in nonalcoholic fatty liver disease. The Journal of Clinical Endocrinology and Metabolism. 2006;**91**(12):4753-4761

[16] Chalasani N, Younossi Z, Lavine JE, Diehl AM, Brunt EM, Cusi K, et al. The diagnosis and management of non-alcoholic fatty liver disease: Practice guideline by the American Association for the Study of Liver Diseases, American College of Gastroenterology, and the American Gastroenterological Association. Hepatology. 2012;**55**(6):2005-2023

[17] Bedossa P. Current histological classification of NAFLD: Strength and limitations. Hepatology International. 2013;**7**(Suppl 2):765-770

[18] Manolio TA, Collins FS. The HapMap and genome-wide association studies in diagnosis and therapy. Annual Review of Medicine. 2009;**60**:443-456

[19] Pandey A, Mann M. Proteomics to study genes and genomes. Nature. 2000;**405**(6788):837-846

[20] Day CP, James OF. Steatohepatitis: A tale of two "hits"? Gastroenterology. 1998;**114**(4): 842-845

[21] Yilmaz Y. Review article: Is non-alcoholic fatty liver disease a spectrum, or are steatosis and non-alcoholic steatohepatitis distinct conditions? Alimentary Pharmacology & Therapeutics. 2012;**36**(9):815-823

[22] Hernaez R. Genetics of non-alcoholic fatty liver disease and associated metabolic disorders. Avances en Diabetología. 2011;**27**(6):186-197

[23] Yuan X, Waterworth D, Perry JR, Lim N, Song K, Chambers JC, et al. Population-based genome-wide association studies reveal six loci influencing plasma levels of liver enzymes. American Journal of Human Genetics. 2008;**83**(4):520-528

[24] Romeo S, Kozlitina J, Xing C, Pertsemlidis A, Cox D, Pennacchio LA, et al. Genetic variation in PNPLA3 confers susceptibility to nonalcoholic fatty liver disease. Nature Genetics. 2008;**40**(12):1461-1465

[25] Krawczyk M, Grunhage F, Zimmer V, Lammert F. Variant adiponutrin (PNPLA3) represents a common fibrosis risk gene: Non-invasive elastography-based study in chronic liver disease. Journal of Hepatology. 2011;**55**(2):299-306

[26] Sookoian S, Pirola CJ. Meta-analysis of the influence of I148M variant of patatin-like phospholipase domain containing 3 gene (PNPLA3) on the susceptibility and histological severity of nonalcoholic fatty liver disease. Hepatology. 2011;**53**(6):1883-1894

[27] Chalasani N, Guo X, Loomba R, Goodarzi MO, Haritunians T, Kwon S, et al. Genome-wide association study identifies variants associated with histologic features of nonalcoholic fatty liver disease. Gastroenterology. 2010;**139**(5):1567-1576 76 e1-6

[28] Speliotes EK, Yerges-Armstrong LM, Wu J, Hernaez R, Kim LJ, Palmer CD, et al. Genome-wide association analysis identifies variants associated with nonalcoholic fatty liver disease that have distinct effects on metabolic traits. PLoS Genetics. 2011;**7**(3):e1001324

[29] Chambers JC, Zhang W, Sehmi J, Li X, Wass MN, Van der Harst P, et al. Genome-wide association study identifies loci influencing concentrations of liver enzymes in plasma. Nature Genetics. 2011;**43**(11):1131-1138

[30] Kozlitina J, Smagris E, Stender S, Nordestgaard BG, Zhou HH, Tybjaerg-Hansen A, et al. Exome-wide association study identifies a TM6SF2 variant that confers susceptibility to nonalcoholic fatty liver disease. Nature Genetics. 2014;**46**(4):352-356

[31] Palmer ND, Musani SK, Yerges-Armstrong LM, Feitosa MF, Bielak LF, Hernaez R, et al. Characterization of European ancestry nonalcoholic fatty liver disease-associated variants in individuals of African and Hispanic descent. Hepatology. 2013;**58**(3):966-975

[32] Anstee QM, Day CP. The genetics of nonalcoholic fatty liver disease: Spotlight on PNPLA3 and TM6SF2. Seminars in Liver Disease. 2015;**35**(3):270-290

[33] Pirola CJ, Sookoian S. The dual and opposite role of the TM6SF2-rs58542926 variant in protecting against cardiovascular disease and conferring risk for nonalcoholic fatty liver: A meta-analysis. Hepatology. 2015;**62**(6):1742-1756

[34] Bernstein BE, Meissner A, Lander ES. The mammalian epigenome. Cell. 2007;**128**(4):669-681

[35] Lee JH, Friso S, Choi SW. Epigenetic mechanisms underlying the link between non-alcoholic fatty liver diseases and nutrition. Nutrients. 2014;**6**(8):3303-3325

[36] Wruck W, Graffmann N, Kawala MA, Adjaye J. Concise review: Current status and future directions on research related to nonalcoholic fatty liver disease. Stem Cells. 2017;**35**(1):89-96

[37] Moleres A, Campion J, Milagro FI, Marcos A, Campoy C, Garagorri JM, et al. Differential DNA methylation patterns between high and low responders to a weight loss intervention in overweight or obese adolescents: The EVASYON study. The FASEB Journal. 2013;**27**(6):2504-2512

[38] Baffy G. MicroRNAs in nonalcoholic fatty liver disease. Journal of Clinical Medicine. 2015;**4**(12):1977-1988

[39] Cermelli S, Ruggieri A, Marrero JA, Ioannou GN, Beretta L. Circulating microRNAs in patients with chronic hepatitis C and non-alcoholic fatty liver disease. PLoS One. 2011;**6**(8):e23937

[40] Pirola CJ, Fernandez Gianotti T, Castano GO, Mallardi P, San Martino J, Mora Gonzalez Lopez Ledesma M, et al. Circulating microRNA signature in non-alcoholic fatty liver disease: From serum non-coding RNAs to liver histology and disease pathogenesis. Gut 2015;**64**(5):800-812

[41] Starmann J, Falth M, Spindelbock W, Lanz KL, Lackner C, Zatloukal K, et al. Gene expression profiling unravels cancer-related hepatic molecular signatures in steatohepatitis but not in steatosis. PLoS One. 2012;**7**(10):e46584

[42] Yoneda M, Endo H, Mawatari H, Nozaki Y, Fujita K, Akiyama T, et al. Gene expression profiling of non-alcoholic steatohepatitis using gene set enrichment analysis. Hepatology Research. 2008;**38**(12):1204-1212

[43] Arendt BM, Comelli EM, Ma DW, Lou W, Teterina A, Kim T, et al. Altered hepatic gene expression in nonalcoholic fatty liver disease is associated with lower hepatic n-3 and n-6 polyunsaturated fatty acids. Hepatology. 2015;**61**(5):1565-1578

[44] Clarke JD, Novak P, Lake AD, Shipkova P, Aranibar N, Robertson D, et al. Characterization of hepatocellular carcinoma related genes and metabolites in human nonalcoholic fatty liver disease. Digestive Diseases and Sciences. 2014;**59**(2):365-374

[45] Lake AD, Novak P, Fisher CD, Jackson JP, Hardwick RN, Billheimer DD, et al. Analysis of global and absorption, distribution, metabolism, and elimination gene expression in the progressive stages of human nonalcoholic fatty liver disease. Drug Metabolism and Disposition. 2011;**39**(10):1954-1960

[46] Moylan CA, Pang H, Dellinger A, Suzuki A, Garrett ME, Guy CD, et al. Hepatic gene expression profiles differentiate presymptomatic patients with mild versus severe non-alcoholic fatty liver disease. Hepatology. 2014;**59**(2):471-482

[47] Murphy SK, Yang H, Moylan CA, Pang H, Dellinger A, Abdelmalek MF, et al. Relationship between methylome and transcriptome in patients with nonalcoholic fatty liver disease. Gastroenterology. 2013;**145**(5):1076-1087

[48] Lefebvre P, Lalloyer F, Bauge E, Pawlak M, Gheeraert C, Dehondt H, et al. Interspecies NASH disease activity whole-genome profiling identifies a fibrogenic role of PPARalpha-regulated dermatopontin. JCI Insight. 2017;**2**(13):e92264

[49] Younossi ZM, Baranova A, Ziegler K, Del Giacco L, Schlauch K, Born TL, et al. A genomic and proteomic study of the spectrum of nonalcoholic fatty liver disease. Hepatology. 2005;**42**(3):665-674

[50] Bell LN, Theodorakis JL, Vuppalanchi R, Saxena R, Bemis KG, Wang M, et al. Serum proteomics and biomarker discovery across the spectrum of nonalcoholic fatty liver disease. Hepatology. 2010;**51**(1):111-120

[51] Verma S, Jensen D, Hart J, Mohanty SR. Predictive value of ALT levels for non-alcoholic steatohepatitis (NASH) and advanced fibrosis in non-alcoholic fatty liver disease (NAFLD). Liver International. 2013;**33**(9):1398-1405

[52] Choe YG, Jin W, Cho YK, Chung WG, Kim HJ, Jeon WK, et al. Apolipoprotein B/AI ratio is independently associated with non-alcoholic fatty liver disease in nondiabetic subjects. Journal of Gastroenterology and Hepatology. 2013;**28**(4):678-683

[53] Gray J, Chattopadhyay D, Beale GS, Patman GL, Miele L, King BP, et al. A proteomic strategy to identify novel serum biomarkers for liver cirrhosis and hepatocellular cancer in individuals with fatty liver disease. BMC Cancer. 2009;**9**:271

[54] Rodriguez-Suarez E, Duce AM, Caballeria J, Martinez Arrieta F, Fernandez E, Gomara C, et al. Non-alcoholic fatty liver disease proteomics. Proteomics. Clinical Applications. 2010;**4**(4):362-371

[55] Sirota JC, McFann K, Targher G, Johnson RJ, Chonchol M, Jalal DI. Elevated serum uric acid levels are associated with non-alcoholic fatty liver disease independently of metabolic syndrome features in the United States: Liver ultrasound data from the National Health and nutrition examination survey. Metabolism. 2013;**62**(3):392-399

[56] Yoneda M, Mawatari H, Fujita K, Iida H, Yonemitsu K, Kato S, et al. High-sensitivity C-reactive protein is an independent clinical feature of nonalcoholic steatohepatitis (NASH) and also of the severity of fibrosis in NASH. Journal of Gastroenterology. 2007; **42**(7):573-582

[57] Yu C, Xu C, Xu L, Yu J, Miao M, Li Y. Serum proteomic analysis revealed diagnostic value of hemoglobin for nonalcoholic fatty liver disease. Journal of Hepatology. 2012;**56**(1):241-247

[58] Kamada Y, Akita M, Takeda Y, Yamada S, Fujii H, Sawai Y, et al. Serum fucosylated haptoglobin as a novel diagnostic biomarker for predicting hepatocyte ballooning and nonalcoholic steatohepatitis. PLoS One. 2013;**8**(6):e66328

[59] Yoneda M, Uchiyama T, Kato S, Endo H, Fujita K, Yoneda K, et al. Plasma Pentraxin3 is a novel marker for nonalcoholic steatohepatitis (NASH). BMC Gastroenterology. 2008;**8**:53

[60] Kwak MS, Kim D, Chung GE, Kang SJ, Park MJ, Kim YJ, et al. Serum bilirubin levels are inversely associated with nonalcoholic fatty liver disease. Clinical and Molecular Hepatology. 2012;**18**(4):383-390

[61] Kaneda H, Hashimoto E, Yatsuji S, Tokushige K, Shiratori K. Hyaluronic acid levels can predict severe fibrosis and platelet counts can predict cirrhosis in patients with nonalcoholic fatty liver disease. Journal of Gastroenterology and Hepatology. 2006;**21**(9): 1459-1465

[62] Yoneda M, Mawatari H, Fujita K, Yonemitsu K, Kato S, Takahashi H, et al. Type IV collagen 7s domain is an independent clinical marker of the severity of fibrosis in patients with nonalcoholic steatohepatitis before the cirrhotic stage. Journal of Gastroenterology. 2007;**42**(5):375-381

[63] Gabrielli GB, Capra F, Casaril M, Corrocher R, Colombari R, De Sandre G. Serum laminin P1 in chronic viral hepatitis: Correlations with liver histological activity and diagnostic value. Clinica Chimica Acta. 1996;**252**(2):171-180

[64] Krishnan A, Li X, Kao WY, Viker K, Butters K, Masuoka H, et al. Lumican, an extracellular matrix proteoglycan, is a novel requisite for hepatic fibrosis. Laboratory Investigation. 2012;**92**(12):1712-1725

[65] D'Amico F, Consolo M, Amoroso A, Skarmoutsou E, Mauceri B, Stivala F, et al. Liver immunolocalization and plasma levels of MMP-9 in non-alcoholic steatohepatitis (NASH) and hepatitis C infection. Acta Histochemica. 2010;**112**(5):474-481

[66] Wanninger J, Walter R, Bauer S, Eisinger K, Schaffler A, Dorn C, et al. MMP-9 activity is increased by adiponectin in primary human hepatocytes but even negatively correlates with serum adiponectin in a rodent model of non-alcoholic steatohepatitis. Experimental and Molecular Pathology. 2011;**91**(2):603-607

[67] Haukeland JW, Damas JK, Konopski Z, Loberg EM, Haaland T, Goverud I, et al. Systemic inflammation in nonalcoholic fatty liver disease is characterized by elevated levels of CCL2. Journal of Hepatology. 2006;**44**(6):1167-1174

[68] Alkhouri N, Lopez R, Berk M, Feldstein AE. Serum retinol-binding protein 4 levels in patients with nonalcoholic fatty liver disease. Journal of Clinical Gastroenterology. 2009;**43**(10):985-989

[69] Graham TE, Yang Q, Bluher M, Hammarstedt A, Ciaraldi TP, Henry RR, et al. Retinol-binding protein 4 and insulin resistance in lean, obese, and diabetic subjects. The New England Journal of Medicine. 2006;**354**(24):2552-2563

[70] Christou GA, Tselepis AD, Kiortsis DN. The metabolic role of retinol binding protein 4: An update. Hormone and Metabolic Research. 2012;**44**(1):6-14

Chapter 2

Molecular Basis for Pathogenesis of Steatohepatitis: Contemporary Understanding and New Insights

Om Parkash and Subha Saeed

Additional information is available at the end of the chapter

http://dx.doi.org/10.5772/intechopen.71405

Abstract

Nonalcoholic fatty liver disease (NAFLD) is characterized by a broad spectrum of clinical and histological presentations, ranging anywhere from simple steatosis to steatohepatitis. Of the patients with NAFLD, only a small fraction goes on to develop inflammation and fibrosis (i.e. NASH). Hence, understanding the underlying molecular mechanisms, which play part in progression of NAFLD and determine the disease severity, is extremely important. Almost two decades ago, Day and colleagues first described the "two-hit hypothesis" to explain progression of NAFLD. However, since then, the advances in field of molecular research have identified that NAFLD development and progression involves complex interplay of numerous determinants, including gut-derived signals, endoplasmic reticulum stress, adipose-derived adipokines, nutritional factors, hormonal imbalances and components of innate immunity which act in concert on genetically predisposed individuals to induce liver inflammation. This chapter reviews the different players of this "multiple-hit model".

Keywords: NAFLD, NASH, molecular basis, "multiple-hit model", steatohepatitis

1. Introduction

Nonalcoholic fatty liver disease (NAFLD) encompasses a broad spectrum of clinical and histo-pathological presentations, ranging from simple steatosis to nonalcoholic steatohepatitis (NASH), the latter being characterized by inflammation, macrovesicular steatosis and apoptosis, with or without fibrosis. NAFLD can further progress to liver fibrosis, cirrhosis and hepatocellular carcinoma (HCC) [1]. The prevalence of NAFLD in Western countries ranges from 30–46% [2], whereas in Asian populations, it is about 15% [3]. About 30% of patients with NAFLD may have NASH [4].

Regarding progression of NASH to cirrhosis, estimated 10% of patients with NASH can progress to decompensated liver disease over 10 years and about 25% of patients develop cirrhosis over a span of 9 years [5]. It is very important to understand and uncover the underlying molecular mechanisms which explain the variable incidence and severity of steatohepatitis in only few patients with NAFLD, while most patients with steatosis never progress to steatohepatitis [6]. After Day and Colleagues first described "two-hit" model for pathogenesis of steatohepatitis in 1998, wherein steatosis ("first hit") progresses to steatohepatitis due to rampant lipid peroxidation in liver ("second hit") [7], recent advances in field of molecular research have identified numerous other culprits, collectively summed up in "multiple-hit" hypothesis [8]. The "multiple-hit" hypothesis examines multiple insults which act collectively and in-parallel on genetically predisposed individuals to induce development of NAFLD and expedite progression to further adverse pathologies. This chapter provides a review of literature for multiple culprits identified in development of NAFLD and NASH.

2. Development of hepatic steatosis

Several mechanisms are involved in development of hepatic steatosis [9–11], including increased fatty acid supply due to increased lipogenesis from both visceral and subcutaneous adipose tissue, increased dietary intake of fats, increased de novo hepatic lipogenesis, decreased free fatty acid oxidation, and decreased secretion of VLDL from liver. Increased free fatty acid delivery to liver and elevated *de novo* lipogenesis are major contributors to fatty acid accumulation in NAFLD.

Elevated hepatic *de novo* lipogenesis may be due to activation by transcription factors such as *SREBP-1*(activated by Insulin, regulated via *Insulin Receptor Substrate* (IRS) and maintains cellular cholesterol homeostasis), *ChREBP* (activated by glucose and increased hepatic *de novo* lipogenesis) and *PPAR-*γ. Studies have demonstrated that *de novo* lipogenesis in liver is elevated in insulin-resistant state and NAFLD [12, 13].

2.1. Lipoapoptosis: free fatty acids and cholesterol

Free fatty acid and Cholesterol are considered main players in lipotoxicity. Increased concentration of serum free fatty acids (16 Carbons and more; saturated or unsaturated) are seen in patients with NAFLD [14]. Apoptosis of hepatocytes, which is morphologic and pathologic feature of human NASH, is partly due to free fatty acids, as explained below.

Hepatocytes can undergo apoptosis via extrinsic pathway (activated by FAS ligand and tumor necrosis factor related apoptosis-inducing ligands) or intrinsic pathway (activated by intracellular stress of membrane-bound organelle, such as mitochondria, endoplasmic reticulum and mitochondria) [15]. Free fatty acids can induce apoptosis via following mechanisms, as demonstrated in **Figure 1**:

- *Mitochondrial pathway* [16] (palmitic acid and stearic acid activate intrinsic apoptotic pathway via C-jun N-terminal kinase and Bim, leading to Bax activation, mitochondrial permeabilization, release of cytochrome c, and activation of Caspase 3 and 7),

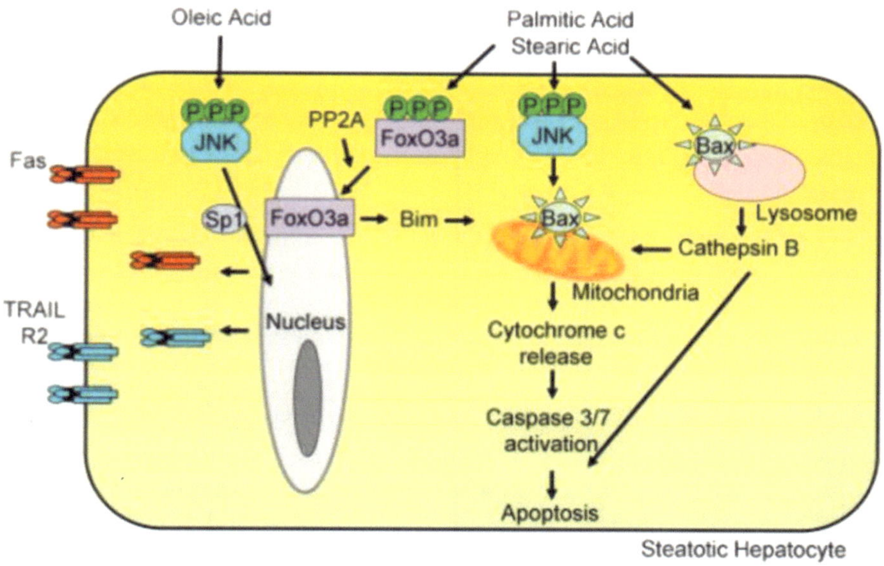

Figure 1. The figure demonstrates different mechanisms by which fatty acids impart lipotoxicity to hepatocytes (copyright © 2008 Georg Thieme Verlag KG) [15] (permission requested from Thieme publications).

- *Induction of Bim expression* [17] (palmitic acid and stearic acid can activate transcription factor FoxO3a, which further induces expression of pro-apoptotic protein Bim),
- *Lysosomal pathway* [18, 19]: Oleic acid and palmitic acid activate Bax which trans-locates to lysosomes, increases the permeability of lysosomes and causes release of cathepsin B, which further increase permeability of mitochondria and activates Caspases. Furthermore, Lysosomal permeabilization is also associated with activation of NF-κB, which results in generation of tumor necrosis factor-α (TNF-α) in hepatocytes,
- *Endoplasmic Reticulum* [20]:Palmitic acid and stearic acid lead to activation of Endoplasmic reticulum (ER) stress pathway, which can lead to apoptosis, as explained later,
- *C-Jun N-Terminal Kinase:* JNK belongs to family of intracellular mitogen-activated protein (MAP). The murine dietary models of obesity were associated with increased activation of JNK in liver [21]. JNK leads to activation of pro-apoptotic protein Bax [22] while it inactivates anti-apoptotic protein, Bcl-2 [23]
- *Death Receptors*: Tumor Necrosis Factor Receptors, TNFR-1 and TNFR-2, and Fas are implicated in pathogenesis of steatohepatitis [24]. Obesity, being a chronic inflammatory state [25], is characterized by infiltration of adipose tissue by macrophages which release of inflammatory mediators, including TNF-α [26], with increased levels of TNF-α being observed in obesity. Upon activation by TNF-α, TNFR-1 activates NF-κB which leads to activation of pro-inflammatory genes and further apoptosis, if NF-κB mediated survival signals are inhibited. TNF-α can also lead to JNK activation, which can also lead to apoptosis if its activation is sustained [15].

Fas is expressed on hepatocytes and upon binding by Fas ligand, it signals apoptotic cell death [15]. In dietary murine models, such as methionine and choline-deficient diet and high sucrose diet, steatosis is accompanied by increased expression of hepatic Fas [27], and increase in Fas expression confers increased Fas ligand-mediated apoptosis. Also, Mono-unsaturated fatty acid, oleic acid, under the transcriptional control of JNK, increases the expression of Fas and TRAIL-R2 on hepatocytes [15]. This is another mechanism by which fatty acids impart sensitivity to death receptor mediated extrinsic pathway of apoptosis,

- *Ceramide*: Ceramides are composed of sphingosine and fatty acid, and availability of long chain fatty acids is a rate limiting step in synthesis of ceramide in ER [28]. In nutritional obesity with associated elevation of palmitic acid and stearic acid, excess synthesis of ceramide is possible. Palmitic acid and stearic acid-induced *de novo* ceramide synthesis in hematopoietic precursor cell line is associated with apoptosis. However, more studies are needed to highlight the exact contribution of ceramide to wide spectrum of NAFLD pathologies [29]
- *Toll-Like Receptors*: toll-like receptors (TLR) are family of pattern recognition receptors that respond to microbial pathogens by activating innate arm of immune system [15]. Palmitic acid activates TLR4, leading to activation of NK-κB. This leads to upregulation of its target genes- i.e. TNF-α and Interleukin-6 (IL-6)- in macrophages and adipocytes [30]. When a high-fat diet is fed to mice lacking TLR4, there is a lack of inflammatory gene expression induction by high-fat diet, pointing towards the role of TLR4 in hepatic inflammation seen in NASH [31].
- *Oxidative Stress*: Enhanced mitochondrial and microsomal fatty acid β oxidation and cytochrome P450 (CYP2E1) induction can lead to oxidative stress via generation of Reactive Oxygen species (ROS), as observed in human models of steatohepatitis [15, 32]. 4-hydroxy-2-noneal (HNE) and Thiobarbituric acid reacting substrate (TBARS), both markers of lipid peroxidation, are increased in patients with NAFLD and NASH [33, 34]. Thus, oxidative stress may contribute towards development of steatosis and steatohepatitis.
- *Long chain poly unsaturated fatty acids* (*LCPUFA*): Oxidative stress leads to depletion of n-3 LCPUFA (e.g Eicosapentaenoic acid, *EPA*, and docosahexaenoic Acid, *DHA*) due to increased peroxidation or defective desaturation processes. Depletion of n-3 LCPUFA leads to upregulation of lipogenic and glycogenic effects from SREBP-1c and down-regulation of fatty acid oxidation effects from peroxisome proliferator activated receptor-α (PPAR-α), ultimately promoting hepatic steatosis [35]. In addition, depletion of LCPUFA can also lead to insulin resistance due to disturbance in membrane mediated processes such as insulin signaling [36]. From dietary prospective, a study aimed at assessing the influence of high-fat diet on $\Delta5$ and $\Delta6$ desaturase enzymes involved in LCPUFA formation, found that HFD lead to enhanced oxidative stress and macrovesicular steatosis, with diminution in desaturase activity and hence, depletion of LCPUFA [37].

The role of cholesterol in lipoapoptosis requires special mention. In an analysis conducted on human liver samples, subjects with NAFLD and NASH exhibited almost a 2-fold increase in free cholesterol, as compared to controls [38]. Furthermore, in a study to evaluate the effect of dietary free cholesterol loading in rodents, rats fed high cholesterol diet developed microvesicular steatosis and were sensitized to apoptotic effect of TNF-α, which may explain the lipoapoptosis due to cholesterol [39].

2.2. Triglycerides

Triglycerides are the main lipids stored in liver of patients with hepatic steatosis and recent studies suggest that triglycerides may in fact have protective functions. Diacylglycerol acyltransferase 1 and 2 (DGAT) catalyze final step in triglyceride synthesis. In a model of diet-induced obesity, mice with over-expression of DGAT1 in adipocytes and macrophages were protected from macrophage activation and accumulation in white adipose tissue, and from systemic inflammation and insulin resistance [9, 40]. In another study, DGAT2 antisense oligonucleotides lead to inhibition of triglycerides synthesis which improved liver steatosis but worsened liver damage, further strengthening the notion that liver triglycerides are protective in nature [41]. Thus, in summary, accumulation of triglycerides in liver might not actually be a pathology but in fact, an adaptive, beneficial response in situations where hepatocytes are exposed to toxic triglyceride metabolites and fatty acid excess due to increased caloric consumption [9, 42].

2.3. Inflammation leads to Steatosis or vice versa: chicken or the egg?

- Treatment with anti-TNF antibody and metformin (an anti-diabetic drug that inhibits hepatic TNFα expression) in ob/ob mice (the laboratory model of nonalcoholic fatty liver disease) showed marked improvement in hepatic steatosis [43, 44].
- In patients with alcoholic steatosis, treatment with anti-TNF antibody can improve hepatic steatosis [45].
- Similarly, loss of Kupffer cells lead to decreased production of anti-inflammatory cytokine (IL-10), which lead to hepatic steatosis [46].

The above examples support the notion that Inflammation activates stress response in hepatocytes, which leads to lipid accumulation. In fact, hepatic steatosis may be considered a *"bystander phenomenon"* following inflammatory attacks. It may be a possibility that inflammation proceeds steatosis in NASH and, benign and non-progressive simple steatosis and NASH are different disease entities altogether [9].

2.4. Insulin resistance in NAFLD

NAFLD is strongly associated with hepatic and adipose tissue insulin resistance, as well as reduced whole body insulin sensitivity [47]. Different underlying molecular mechanisms have been identified which account for insulin resistance [8]:

1. Serine phosphorylation of insulin receptor substrate (IRS) by inflammatory signals, such *as c-jun N-terminal protein kinase 1* (JNK) or *inhibitor of nuclear factor-jB kinase-b* (IKKb) [48]
2. *Activation of nuclear factor kappa B* (NF-κB) and *Suppressors of cytokine signaling* (SOCS) [49]

Insulin Resistance would mean that ability of Insulin to suppress lipolysis has been supressed, leading to increased delivery of free fatty acids to liver [50]. The free fatty acid can further exacerbate hepatic insulin resistance by causing translocation of PKC-γ isoform from cytosol to the membrane where it impairs hepatic *insulin receptor substrate* (IRS)-associated phosphatidylinositol activity [51].

2.4.1. Oxidative stress and insulin resistance

Prolonged excess oxidative load in steatosis, due to carbohydrates and lipids, leads to redox disequilibrium characterized by lower than normal hepatic anti-oxidative potential, for example, decreased hepatic glutathione (GSH) and reduced superoxide dismutase (SOD) activity, which further triggers insulin resistance (IR) [52]. This is validated by a data from study where increased reactive oxygen species (ROS) in 3T3-L1 cultured pre-adipocytes preceded the onset of Insulin resistance [53], by molecular mechanisms listed above. The insulin resistance due to exacerbated hepatic oxidative stress can in turn lead to upregulation of pro-oxidative CYP2E1 expression, the response which is normally attenuated by repressive effects of Insulin on CYP2E1 expression [54]. Thus, there is increasing evidence for positive reinforcement and interdependency between oxidative stress and insulin resistance in patients with Hepatic steatosis [52].

Thus, due to impairment in IRS activity and further down-regulation of IRS due to insulin resistance, SREBP is unregulated and over-expressed, leading to increased hepatic *de novo* lipogenesis [55]. Insulin Resistance, due to its ability to induce lipotoxicity, oxidative stress and inflammatory cascade, may be one of the "multiple hit" in pathogenesis of NAFLD and progression towards NASH [8, 56].

3. The gut-derived factors

The gut microbiota is implicated in the pathogenesis and progression of NAFLD, through so-called gut-liver axis [8]. A study aimed at analyzing human gut microbiome recognized different "enterotypes" [57] and "obese microbiome", which has an ability to harvest increased amount of energy from diet, has been demonstrated in obese mice [58]. In fact, colonization of germ-free mice with "obese microbiome" leads to greater increase in total body fat as compared to colonization with "lean microbiome" [58]. The **Figure 2** summarizes the role of gut-liver axis and adipose tissue in pathogenesis of NAFLD.

The liver receives more than 50% of its blood supply from splanchnic circulation [8], and hence, it is always exposed to gut-derived toxins. The ability of gut-derived factors like lipopolysaccharide (LPS) to flow in portal vein requires intestinal permeability, which in NAFLD is due to disrupted intercellular tight junctions in the intestine [59]. In Murine models of NAFLD, intestinal mucosa has bacterial overgrowth with increased intestinal permeability and concurrent reduction in expression of tight junction proteins [60]. Consequentially, plasma endotoxin levels are significantly high in patients with NAFLD and NASH [61], and high-fat diet is associated with 2–3 fold increase in plasma LPS levels [62]. LPS may act as a ligand for TLR with consequent activation of inflammatory cascade, including stress- and mitogen-activated protein kinases-JNK (explained later), p38, Interferon regulatory factors 3 and nuclear factor-jB – each having

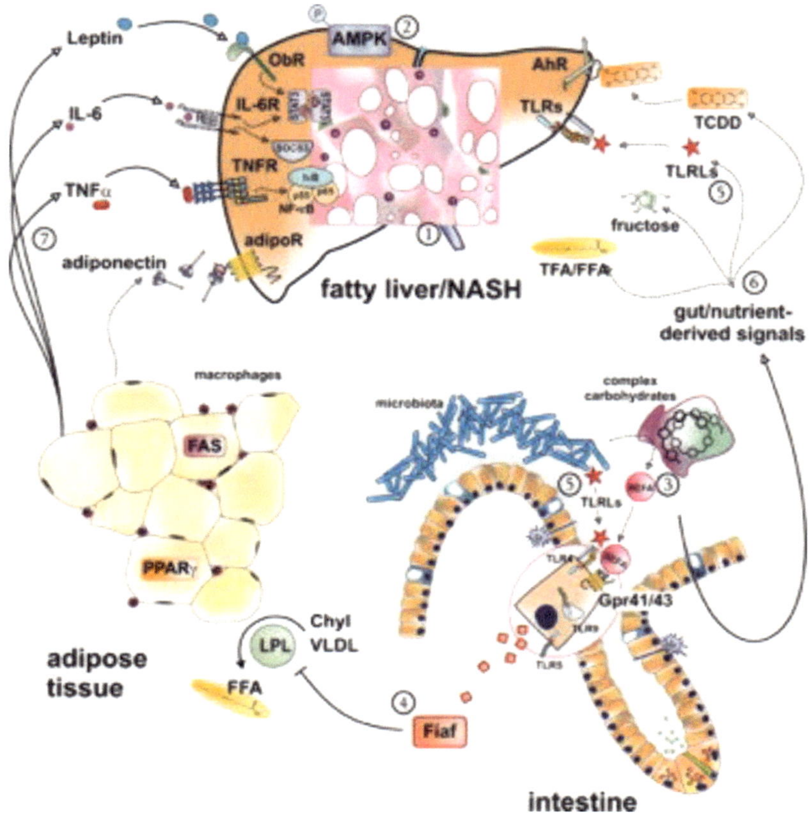

Figure 2. "The multiple parallel hits model. Lipotoxicity: (1) a liver loaded with lipids consisting primarily of trigylcerides might reflect a benign process because triglycerides might exert mostly protective effects. Furthermore, hyperleptinemia leads to oxidation of hepatic lipids, thereby also protecting this organ from lipotoxicity. When the capacity of peripheral and central organs of detoxifying "aggressive lipids" fails, lipotoxic attack of the liver might begin. Inflammation may precede steatosis in NASH. Gut-derived signals: Many signals beyond endotoxin might affect hepatic steatosis and inflammation. Several pathways have been identified how the gut microbiota might influence host energy metabolism: (2) Absence of the microbiota in germ-free mice correlates with increased activity of phosphorylated AMPK in the liver and the muscle (not shown). (3) Some of the breakdown products of polysaccharides are metabolized to SCFAs. SCFAs such as propionate and acetate are ligands for the G protein-coupled receptors Gpr41 and Gpr43. Shortage of SCFAs might allow the evolution of systemic inflammatory events. Such mechanisms elegantly combine diet, microbiota, and the epithelial cell as "nutrient sensor." (4) The microbiota decreases epithelial expression of fasting-induced adipocyte factor (Fiaf), which functions as a circulating lipoprotein lipase (LPL) inhibitor and therefore is an important regulator of peripheral fat storage. (5) Several TLRs, such as TLR5 or TLR9, are not only able to affect microbiota but also to regulate metabolism, systemic inflammation, and insulin resistance, thus highlighting the role of the innate immune system in metabolic inflammation as observed in NASH. (6) Various nutrients such as trans fatty acids (TFAs), fructose or aryl hydrocarbon receptor (AhR) ligands such as 2,3,7,8-tetrachlorodibenzodioxin (TCDD) may directly lead to steatosis/liver inflammation. Adipose tissue-derived signals: Signals derived from the adipose tissue beyond toxic lipids might play a central role in NAFLD/NASH. (7) here, adipocytokines such as adiponectin and leptin, certain pro-inflammatory cytokines such as TNFα or IL-6, and others (the death receptor Fas, PPARγ) are of key relevance. The cytokine/adipocytokine milieu might be critical because ob/ob-adiponectin tg mice, although becoming severely obese, are not insulin-resistant. This suggests that in the hierarchy of processes soluble mediators play the central role. Adipose-derived mediators might indeed affect target organs such as the liver, because JNK1 adipose-deficient mice are protected from diet-induced obesity, and experiments have demonstrated that this effect is mediated mainly by IL-6 (a cytokine), which is of key importance in human obesity." [9] (figure and associated caption used after permission from "John Wiley and Sons" [9]).

significant contribution towards insulin resistance, hepatic fat accumulation, obesity and NASH development and progression [63, 64]. Evidently, a continuous infusion of LPS for 4 weeks in mice mimicked high-fat diet phenotype, with noticeable increase in insulin resistance, increased liver triglyceride content and adipose tissue inflammation [62]. Similarly, the use of antibiotics reduced the intensity of inflammation in high-fat diet and ob/ob mice [65].

Another mechanism for gut microbiota to influence the host immune system is via their capacity to digest dietary fibers, such as resistant starch and nonstarch polysaccharide, to short chain fatty acids (SCFAs, mainly propionate, butyrate and acetate), which are absorbed by intestinal epithelium [66]. SCFAs, via their interactions with G protein-coupled receptor 43 (Gpr43), have anti-inflammatory function in various models of human ulcerative colitis [67, 68].

Enteric bacteria also suppress the synthesis of fasting-induced adipocyte factor (Fiaf), resulting in increased lipoprotein lipase activity and increased triglyceride accumulation in the liver [8, 9]. Gut microbiota also produce enzymes which cause the conversion of dietary choline to toxic compounds, particularly methylamines which, in the liver, are transformed to trimethylamine-N-oxide and induce inflammation and liver fibrosis [69]. Intestinal microbiome is a major source for production of hepatotoxic compounds such as alcohol, phenols and ammonia which are delivered to the liver by portal circulation. These compounds activate kupffer cells and stimulate the production of nitric oxide and other inflammatory cytokines [70]. Patients with NASH show abundance of alcohol-producing bacteria as compared to healthy children and children with simple steatosis [71]. This endogenous production of alcohol has a well-established role in generation of ROS and liver inflammation [72].

Furthermore, NLRP6 and NLRP3 inflammasomes, through their production of IL-18, play an important role in modulation of gut microbiota. In different mouse models, inflammasomes deficiency is associated with modifications in configuration of gut microbiota, and exacerbation of hepatic steatosis and inflammation. This is due to increased influx of TLR4 and TLR9 ligands into the portal circulation, leading to enhanced tumor necrosis factor-α (TNF-α) production in liver which leads to NASH progression [73].

3.1. Bile acids

The primary bile acids cholic acid and chenodeoxycholic acid are conjugated to glycine and taken up in distal ileum for transport to the liver [74]. By binding to cellular receptor farnesoid X receptor (FXR) in various organs of the body, bile acids act as signaling molecules to control overall metabolism of the host [75]. Upon activation of FXR by primary bile acids, downstream signals are generated which lead to inhibition of hepatic *de novo* lipogenesis, increased insulin sensitivity and protection of hepatocytes from bile acid-induced cytotoxicity [76]. However, the gut microbiota in distal ileum can deconjugate the bile acids and can further metabolize them to secondary bile acids, and thus, contribute towards obesity by altering lipid metabolism, through changes in bile acid pools and modulation of FXR signaling [74].

3.2. Dietary factors

The recent decades saw a dramatic increase in consumption of trans-fatty acids, and as evident from studies on mice, trans-fatty acids consumption leads to larger liver with NASH-like lesions and Insulin resistance [77]. Similarly, Fructose is a lipogenic, pro-inflammatory dietary factor associated with oxidative stress and upregulation of TNF-α [78], and daily fructose consumption is associated with liver inflammation and fibrosis [79]. Fructose diet can induce oxidative stress and hepatocellular damage by different mechanisms, including induction of protein fructosylation which activates SREBP and generates reactive oxygen species (ROS) [80]. Also fructose phosphorylation leads to depletion of ATP, which stimulates increased uric acid synthesis which in turn stimulates production of ROS [81]. Lastly fructose can induce mitochondrial disturbance which lead to disequilibrium between *De novo Lipogenesis* and VLDL, which promotes alteration of respiratory chain and uncoupling of oxidative phosphorylation with excess ROS production [82, 83].

Another receptor, aryl hydrocarbon receptor (AhR), is a ligand activated transcription factor which is activated by many constituents of our diet such as indolo-(3,2-b)-carbazole and 3,3′-diindolylmethane (metabolized from indole 2-carbinol), or flavonoids, and this pathway plays an important role in inflammation [84]. This is evident in transgenic mice with constitutively activated AhR as they develop spontaneous hepatic steatosis and increased hepatic oxidative stress [85].

Studies show that Low-Calorie, Low-carbohydrate soy-containing diet and Mediterranean diet rich in antioxidants and polyunsaturated fatty acids of n-3 series are known to be protective in reducing hepatic steatosis [86].

4. Adipose tissue-derived signal

Adipose tissue, with its ability to generate cytokines and adipocytokines, can be classified as a complex endocrine and immune organ which mediates different metabolic, immunological and inflammatory responses.

4.1. Adiponectin

Adiponectin is an anti-inflammatory cytokine with anti-lipogenic effects which protect non-adipocyte tissue, such as liver, from lipid accumulation [87]. Reduced levels of adiponectin are seen in conditions associated with development of NAFLD, namely obesity [88] and insulin resistance [89]. Hence, adiponectin levels are inversely related to visceral obesity and insulin resistance, and weight loss is an inducer of adiponectin synthesis [90]. The levels of adiponectin are significantly reduced in patients with NASH as compared to simple steatosis [91]. Thus adiponectin protects the liver against steatosis.

By activating cyclic-AMP dependent protein kinase (AMPK), adiponectin opposes fatty acid synthesis and promotes mitochondrial β-oxidation [92]. The anti-inflammatory effects of adiponectin are due to its ability to block activation of NF-κB which inhibits the release of pro-inflammatory cytokines such as TNFα and IL-6 [93]. The anti-inflammatory and hepatic lipid modulating effects of adiponectin may also be due to activation of peroxisome proliferator activated receptor-α (PPAR-α), as pharmacological treatment with PPAR-α agonist reverses experimental steatohepatitis [94]. Furthermore, PPAR-γ agonist, such as thiazolidinedione, stimulate adiponectin synthesis, and latter activates PPAR-α [95].

4.2. Leptin

Leptin is a gene product of *ob* gene and is produced by visceral adipocytes [96]. The levels of leptin directly correlate with body fat mass and adipocyte size [97]. Leptin has a potential dual action on NAFLD experimental models, exerting anti-steatotic, and pro-inflammatory/pro-fibrogenic actions [98]. In non-adipose tissue, such as liver, it prevents lipid accumulation by decreasing the expression of SREBP-1. Leptin exerts pro-fibrogenic effects by activating stellate cell in liver through hedgehock [99], mTOR [100] or kupffer cell-mediated TGF-β1 secretion which then activates stellate cell [101]. In mice models of NASH, gut-derived endotoxins can induce hyper-responsiveness to leptin, with subsequent upregulation of CD14 and accelerated fibrosis [102]. Experimental studies have demonstrated that leptin deficiency in mice may lead to hepatic steatosis which can be reversed by leptin replacement. On the other hand, excess leptin contributes towards hepatic inflammation and fibrosis [98]. It may be a possibility that anti-steatosis effects of leptin may predominate in initial stages of NAFLD while pro-inflammatory and pro-fibrotic effects might take over during disease progression phase [103]. However, the exact magnitude of contribution by Leptin towards NAFLD remains to be elucidated.

4.3. IL-6 and TNFα

In severe obesity, adipocytes are major source of IL-6 production, as evident by a study results where IL-6 expression was 100-fold elevated in adipose tissue as compared to liver in obese patients [9]. Similarly, elevated TNF-α production has been observed in cultures of peripheral blood cells collected from obese patients with NASH [104]. These two important pro-inflammatory cytokines are found to be elevated in obese patients and weight loss is associated with dramatic decrease in serum levels of these cytokines [105, 106].

The liver is the target organ for adipose tissue-derived 1 L-6 and TNFα. It is known that high-fat diet, also called "inflammatory diet", stimulates *JNK1* (mitogen-activated protein kinase, associated with apoptosis) signaling in adipocytes, which leads to IL-6 secretion by adipocytes. IL-6 further acts on hepatic cell, leading to hepatic steatosis and hepatic insulin resistance [48]. Continuous exposure to elevated levels of IL-6/TNF-α leads to many of the histological features of NASH such as hepatocyte necrosis and apoptosis, neutrophil chemotaxis and activation of hepatic stellate cells [107]. Also, they caused insulin resistance by upregulating hepatic suppressor of cytokine signaling 3 (SOCS3) [108].

Transcription factor *nuclear factor-jB kinase b* (NF-κB) and its IKK2 subunits is also important mediators of chronic inflammatory states. Persistent activation of NF-κB has been shown in animal models of NAFLD [109] and NASH [110].

4.4. Inflammasomes

Inflammasomes are large caspase-1 –activating multiprotein complexes that sense both endogenous and exogenous danger signals via intracellular NOD-like receptors (NLRs) [111]. Among the three prototypes of inflammasomes, NALP3 is associated with NAFLD and responds to danger signals by activating Caspase 1. Active Caspase-1 promotes cleavage and maturation of pro-inflammatory cytokines, such as IL-1β, IL-18, IL-33, which further promote inflammation [111]. Gut-derived endotoxin and free fatty acid may act as danger associated molecular pattern (DAMP) which may lead to activation of inflammasomes [112].

To validate the role of inflammasomes in NASH, it was seen that there was increased gene expression of inflammasomes in livers of patients with NASH as compared to liver of healthy controls [113]. Furthermore, LPS and saturated fatty acids amplify the expression and activation of inflammasomes, and free fatty acids sensitize the hepatocytes to LPS-induced IL-1β secretion [112]. It was seen observed that saturated fatty acids also directly induce hepatocyte apoptosis and activation of Caspase 8, which triggers the release of danger molecules from hepatocytes [112].

IL-1β induces the suppression of peroxisome proliferator activated receptor-α (PPAR-α), activates the stellate cells to promote fibrosis and promotes TNF-α-induced cell death [114].

5. Toll-like receptors and innate immunity

Toll-like receptors are sensors of microbial and endogenous danger signals which are expressed in innate immune cells and liver parenchyma and contribute towards progression of NASH [90]. Upon activation by gut microbiota-released pathogen- or damage- associated molecular pattern (PAMP and DAMP), downstream signals are activated which lead to progression of NASH. TLR2, TLR4 and TLR9 are most commonly associated with NASH [90].

The gut-derived bacterial endotoxin is brought to liver via portal circulation where they activate the kupffer cell by way of TLR4 receptor complex. This interaction leads to activation of nuclear transcription factors, leading to release of pro-inflammatory mediators such as TNFα which can induce liver injury and fibrosis [115]. The role of TLR4 in pathogenesis of NASH is further supported by study where TLR4-deficient mice, which were fed high fructose diet,were protected from formation of reactive oxygen species, induction of TNFα expression in liver and insulin resistance [116].

TLR9 is located on endoplasmic reticulum and is activated by unmethylated CpG DNA particles that are released from bacteria [90]. It is known that TLR9 is involved in steatohepatitis as TLR9-deficient mice are protected from liver inflammation [114]. In *CDAA diet*-(Choline-deficient amino acid defined diet) induced NASH, translocated bacterial DNA from gut binds to TLR9 receptor on kupffer cell to produce IL-1β which activate hepatic stellate cells to induce liver fibrosis, and also stimulate hepatocytes for lipid accumulation and cell death [114]. The induction of hepatic steatosis is independent of TLR2, however, functional TLR2 receptors are found on kupffer cells which mediate liver inflammation and fibrosis in CDAA diet-induced NASH [117].

Recently, another data that implicated TLR5 in pathogenesis of metabolic syndrome was presented. It was reported that mice deficient in TLR5 developed all features of metabolic syndrome including, hyperphagia, obesity, insulin resistance, pancreatic inflammation and hepatic steatosis. It was proposed that TLR5 altered the gut microbiota and the finding were reproducible when microbiota from TLR5 $^{-/-}$ mice was transferred to healthy mice [118]. However, another study did not find any such results in TLR5-deficient mice [119]. Indeed, more studies are needed to elicit role of TLR5 in steatohepatitis.

6. Endoplasmic reticulum (ER) stress

Endoplasmic reticulum (ER) is an important intracellular organelle involved in production, folding, post-translational modification and trafficking of secretory and membrane proteins. Also present in the ER is endoplasmic reticulum-associated degradation (ERAD) machinery that ensures that misfolded proteins are re-translocated back to cytoplasm for degradation by proteasomes [120]. Thus, ER serves as a quality control checkpoint, allowing only properly folded proteins to be transported to Golgi apparatus [121, 122] (**Figure 3**).

Any event that disturbs ER protein folding capacity- be it due to excessive protein synthesis, accumulation of misfolded proteins, depletion of calcium in ER, disturbance in redox regulation, glucose depletion, viral infection or high-fat diet (saturated fatty acid such as palmitic acid and stearic acid) [123] - leads to induction of evolutionarily conserved ER stress response, known as Unfolded protein response (UPR). The role of sensing ER stress and activating UPR is performed by three ER transmembrane proteins, mentioned as following:

1. RNA-dependent Protein kinase-like ER eukaryotic initiation factor-2α Kinase (PERK)
2. Inositol-requiring ER-to-nucleus signaling protein1 (IRE1) and,
3. Transcription factor 6 (ATF6)

Each of these transmembrane proteins has an ER luminal domain to sense unfolded protein, a transfolded domain for targeting to the ER membrane, and a cytosolic domain to transmit signals to the transcriptional and/or translational apparatus [124]. In an unstressed cell, these ER proteins are maintained in an inactive state via their association with the ER chaperon protein, glucose-regulated protein 78 (GRP78)/Bip [125] and upon ER stress, unfolded/ misfolded proteins accumulation enhances the release of GRP78 from these stress-sensing proteins, leading to respective activation of PERK, ATF6 and IRE1 [126].

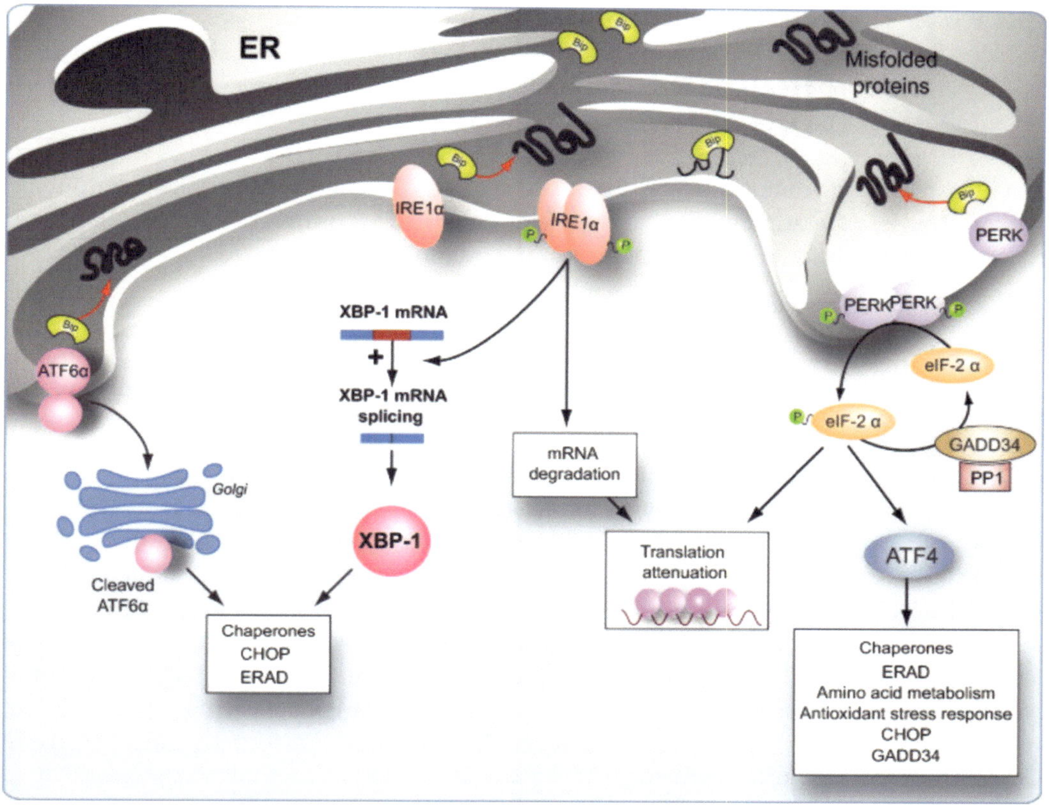

Figure 3. The figure demonstrating the three different pathways of unfolded protein response [135] (https://doi.org/10.1016/j.jhep.2010.11.005) (http://creativecommons.org/licenses/by-nc-nd/4.0/).

Upon activation, PERK, IRE1α and ATF6 induce signal transduction events that attenuate the accumulation of misfolded proteins in the ER by increasing expression of ER chaperons, inhibiting protein load on ER by decreasing mRNA translation, and stimulating retrograde transport of misfolded proteins from ER into cytosol for ubiquination and destruction by a process named ERAD [127]. However, under conditions where ER stress is chronically prolonged and the cell fails to restore homeostatsis in ER, the UPR will initiate cell apoptosis [126].

6.1. Protein kinase RNA-like endoplasmic reticulum kinase (PERK)

Activation of PERK leads to phosphorylation of α-subunit of eukaryotic Initiation Factor 2α (eIF-2α), leading to its inactivation and hence, attenuation of mRNA translation and decreased protein load on the ER [128]. The phosphorylated eIF-2α also causes preferential translation of UPR-dependent genes, such as activation transcription factor 4 (ATF 4). Further, ATF4 induces expression of several genes, including amino acid transporter, chaperons and CHOP [129] (*"C/EBP homologous protein"*, also known *as 'growth arrest and DNA damage* (*GADD 15*)).

CHOP is an ER-derived transcription factor which is an important mediator of ER stress-induced apoptosis, as evident from studies where deletion of CHOP lead to attenuation of hepatocellular apoptosis in alcohol- and cholestasis-induced liver disease [130]. Apoptosis-relevant targets of the CHOP transcription factor include:

1. *GADD34* [131]: promotes dephosphorylation of eIF2α,thus reversing translation inhibition. This leads to accumulation of unfolded proteins in ER compartment, and, simultaneously, permits translation of mRNA encoding pro-apoptotic genes,
2. *DR5*: a caspase activating cell-surface death receptor, and
3. *Ero 1 α* (Endoplasmic Reticulum Oxidoreductase-1): hyperoxdises the ER and also activates the inositol triphosphate receptor (IP_3R), causing excessive transport of Calcium from ER to the mitochondria and thus causing cell death) [132].

CHOP also induces apoptosis via direct inhibition of Bcl-2 transcription [133] and induction of Bim expression [134]. Bcl-2 proteins are localized within the ER membrane and are protective (*anti-apoptotic*) against ER stress. This cytoprotective function is mainly due to the ability of Bcl-2 to lower steady-state levels of ER Ca^{2+} via IP_3Rs. The protective role of Bcl-2 in regulating ER Ca^{2+} can be inhibited by JNK-mediated phosphorylation of Bcl-2. The Phosphorylated Bcl-2 loses its anti-apoptotic function by being unable to bind *pro-apoptotic* "BH_3-only" members of Bcl-2 family (i.e. Bim), leading to increasing calcium release from ER, which is associated with mitochondrial calcium uptake. This leads to increased mitochondrial permeabilization, release of cytochrome C, and hence apoptosis [127]. Calcium release from ER can also activate Caplains, which may further proteolytically activate Caspase-12 to induce apoptosis [135].

6.2. Inositol-requiring ER-to-nucleus signaling protein1 (IRE1)

Accumulation of unfolded proteins in ER leads to activation of IRE1, which further processes an intron from X-box binding protein-1 (XBP-1) mRNA and permits synthesis of XBP-1 protein. XBP-1 binds to promoters of genes involved in UPR (encoding ER chaperons) and ERAD to restore homeostasis and prevent cellular toxicity [127]. Apart from cytoprotective effects, IRE1 can also recruits inflammatory factors (JNK and NF-κB) which induce inflammatory response signaling [136], and apoptotic signal kinase-1 (ASK1) which causes downstream activation of stress kinases Jun-N-terminal Kinase (JNK) and p38 MAPK, that promotes apoptosis [137].

Activated JNK translocate to mitochondria and causes activation of Bim and Inhibition of Bcl-2. Activated JNK also induces the expression of pro-inflammatory genes by phosphorylating transcription factor activating protein-1(AP-1) [138]· Activated p38 MAPK phosphorylates and activates CHOP [127] to causes apoptosis.

6.3. Transcription factor 6 (ATF6)

ATF6 belongs to CREB family of transcription factors. Activation of ATF6 leads to its release from ER membrane, processing in the Golgi and entry into the nucleus. It trans-activates ER stress related genes such as ER chaperones, XBP-1, foldases and CHOP [124].

6.4. Endoplasmic reticulum stress and Steatosis

Hepatocytes, being rich in both smooth and rough EPR, perform diverse metabolic functions, including lipoprotein and very-low-density lipoprotein (VLDL) assembly and secretion, cholesterol biosynthesis and xenobiotic metabolism [121]. The Sterol regulatory element-binding protein (SREBPs) are key regulators of lipid homoeostasis and play crucial role in *de novo* lipogenesis [139], where SREBP-1 regulates fatty acid and triglycerides (TG) metabolism and SREBP-2 controls cholesterol metabolism and low density lipoprotein (LDL) receptor expression [140]. SREBP are transcription factors bound to ER membrane in inactive form and their activity is controlled within ER by interaction of *SREBP-Cleavage Activating Protein* (SCAP) and *Insulin regulated proteins* (Insigs). Insigs cause SREBP-SCAP complex to be retained within the ER and prevents SREBP-1 activation [141]. Under conditions of low sterols, Insigs are dissociated with SCAP, leading to migration of SREBP-SCAP complex to Golgi apparatus, where SREBP is processed to its active form by S1P and S2P [142]. Activated SREBP translocate to nucleus and regulates the various genes involved in lipid metabolism.

However, under ER Stress, rapid activation of precursor form of SREBP-1c and SREBP-1c target genes takes place, even in absence of Insulin [143]. Furthermore, ER stress induces proteolytic activation of SREBPs by increasing turnover of Insigs [142]. Hence, the recent data suggests that ER stress leads to hepatic steatosis by increasing de novo lipogenesis and upregulating the transcription of genes encoding for key lipogenic trans-activators and enzymes [121, 144].

Due to its high capacity for protein synthesis, ER stress plays an important part in mediating pathological changes in various liver diseases [135]. The signaling pathway activated by ER stress are implicated in lipotoxicity, Insulin Resistance, Inflammation and apoptotic cell death which are common to both NAFLD and NASH [123]. The presence of ER stress and activation of UPR in chronic disease (such as NAFLD) suggests that ability to resolve ER stress has been compromised. Inducing ER stress in individuals with genetically ablated eIF2α, IRE1α or ATF6α leads to hepatic steatosis [145], suggesting that steatosis results from impairment in the capacity to oxidize fatty acids and augmented by impaired lipoprotein secretion. Thus, initially UPR aims to prevent steatosis and re-establish *ER homeostasis* after ER stress but selective impairment to the UPR that reduce the ability of UPR to resolve ER stress leads to development and exacerbation of hepatic steatosis. However, further work is needed to investigate this Homeostatic Model hypothesis.

It is now well-established that various arms of UPR and its downstream signaling molecules play role in regulation of lipid metabolism and induction of various hepatic pathologies.

6.4.1. PERK-eIF2α-ATF4 pathway

The PERK-eIF2α-ATF4 pathway is reported to regulate lipogenesis and hepatic steatosis. PERK-dependent signaling has been crucial to sustained expression of lipogenic enzymes such as fatty acid synthase (FAS), ATP-citrate Lyase, and stearoyl-CoA Desaturase-1(SCD1) [146]. Phosphorylated eIF2α (activated form) is associated with enhanced expression of adipogenic nuclear receptor peroxisome proliferator activated receptor γ (PPAR γ) and its upstream regulators, and dephosphorylation of eIF2α using GADD34 leads to diminished hepatosteatosis in animals fed high-fat diet [147]. Furthermore, activated ATF4 increases expression of lipogenic genes, such as PPAR γ, sterol regulatory element-binding protein-1c (SREBP-1c), acetyl-CoA carboxylase (ACC), and FAS, in liver and white adipose tissue. Similarly, ATF4 knockout mice are protected from diet-induced hepatic steatosis [148, 149]. Thus, the current evidence suggests that PERK-eIF2α-ATF4 pathway plays an important role in promoting lipogenesis.

6.4.2. IRE1α-XBP1 pathway

The IRE1α-XBP1 pathway plays an important part in maintenance of hepatic lipid homeostatsis under ER stress and regulation of hepatic VLDL assembly and secretion [150]. IRE1α is also required for efficient synthesis of ApoB-containing lipoproteins [151]. Mice with hepatocyte specific deletion of IREIα show increased hepatic steatosis and reduced plasma lipids under ER stress condition due to altered expression of key metabolic players (such as PPARγ and C/EBPβ) and of enzymes involved in Triglycerides biosynthesis [151]. Thus, these results indicate IRE1α represses lipid accumulation in liver, especially under ER stress condition. However, the deletion of IRE1α leads to loss of this protective role of IRE1α, resulting in unresolved ER stress and hence, hepatic steatosis.

The role of XBP1 in lipogenesis is emphasized in a study where conditional disruption of XBP-1 in the liver of mice lead to reduced plasma level of triglycerides, cholesterol and free fatty acids, possibly due to decreased de novo lipogenesis [152]. XBP1 regulates lipogenesis in hepatocytes by directly binding to promotors of lipogenic genes such as SCD1 (Stearoyl-CoA Desaturase 1), DGAT2 (Diacylglycerol Transferase 2) and ACC2 (Acetyl-CoA carboxylase),thereby activating their transcription [152]. Thus under appropriate conditions, XBP1 promotes lipogenesis and contributes to hepatic lipogenesis.

6.4.3. Transcription factor 6 (ATF6)

ATF6 and SREBP are both ER membrane bound transcription factors, and nuclear ATF6 interacts with nuclear SREBP 2, antagonizing the SREBP2- regulated transcription of lipogenic genes and preventing lipid accumulation in cultures of liver cell [153]. Moreover, ATF2α-knockout mice develop hepatic steatosis in response to ER stress, due to reduced fatty acid oxidation and decreased VLDL secretion [154].

Thus, taken together, all three proximal UPR sensors including PERK, IRE1α and ATF6α, regulate lipid stores in liver but the degree to which the UPR contributes to hepatic steatosis may depend on activation of three proximal UPR sensors relative to each other, coupled with appropriate downstream protein–protein and/or protein-DNA interaction [120].

6.5. Endoplasmic reticulum stress and progression towards NASH

Multiple factors, including but not limited to, insulin action, oxidative stress, cytokine mediated signaling, inflammation, bacterial endotoxin, and excess fatty acids function in concert and interact with UPR to provoke disease progression of NAFLD towards NASH.

6.5.1. ER stress and hepatic inflammation

Several Signaling pathways connect ER stress to hepatic inflammation:

- Reactive oxygen species (ROS)

  Protein folding in ER is intimately linked to generation of ROS, such that each disulfide bond formation during oxidative protein folding leads to production of 1 ROS [155]. An elevated protein folding load, as in ER stress, leads to accumulation of ROS, which may lead to inflammation. In turn, the oxidative stress from ROS can disrupt ER homeostasis and induce ER stress [156].

  However, in an unsurprising adaptive pathway, UPR activates an antioxidant program via transcription factor *Nrf2* (nuclear factor erythroid-derived 2-related factor 2) to prevent accumulation of ROS [157]. *Nrf2* is activated after phosphorylation by PERK pathway of UPR and it regulates the inducible expression of anti-oxidant response element-containing genes [157]. Importantly, Nrf2 deletion results in rapid onset and progression of steatohepatitis in mice provided a methionine choline-deficient (MCD) diet [158]. ATF4, one of the other terminal player of PERK pathway, has also been an important transcription factor in maintenance of adequate Glutathione levels in cells [159]. Thus, PERK arm of UPR and its downstream players are directly related to regulation of anti-oxidant effects. In a recent study, IRE1α-XBP1 branch of UPR was also found linked to anti-oxidant effect, where XBP1 deficiency leads to reduced catalase expression [160].

- NF-κB and JNK

  In response to ER stress, IRE1α binds to adaptor protein tumor-necrosis factor α (TNF-α) receptor-associated factor 2 (TRAF2). IRE1α-TRAF2 complex activates NF-κB and JNK, both of which induce production of Pro-inflammatory cytokines, such as C-reactive protein (CRP), amyloid P-component, fibrinogen, and interleukin-6 (IL-6) [161].

  The UPR-mediated signaling can lead to activation of NF-κB not only via IRE1α but also via PERK [162] and/or ATF6 pathway [163]. Activation of NF-κB has been detected in steatohepatitis induced by MCD diet, however, the exact mechanism about how ER stress-induced signaling involving NK-κB and JNK might regulate inflammation, cell survival and apoptosis in NAFLD is still unknown.

- PKR (double-stranded RNA-activated Protein Kinase)

  PKR is an interferon-induced Serine/threonine protein kinase, activated by dsRNA, and is capable of activating NF-κB and eIF2α in response to dsRNA and oxidative stress, respectively [164]. PKR activity is increased in adipose tissue and liver of murine model of obesity [165]. With its ability to respond to pathogens, nutrients and organelle stress, PKR appears to be core component of inflammatory and immune pathways. However, depending on which key factor is activated downstream, that is, either NF-κB (pro-apoptotic) or eIF2α (anti-apoptotic), PKR may "serve as molecular clock to time the sequential events of survival and death" [166]. In summary, PKR affirms the complexity of UPR signaling and its downstream outcomes [120].

- CREBH

  CREBH is a transcription factor belonging to CREB/ATF family of transcription factor and is required for liver synthesis of Amyloid P-component and CRP [167]. CREBH is activated via RIP process (Regulated Intramembrane Proteolysis: release and transport of ER resident protein from the ER membrane to Golgi for processing) upon ER stress. Other than ER stress, TNFα, Interleukin 6 (IL6) and lipoprotein LPS also induce expression of CREBH [168]. This makes room for another revelation: ER stress in the liver may be linked to systemic inflammation via the RIP- mediated mobilization of CREBH [120].

6.5.2. ER stress and apoptosis

Apoptosis is an important component of disease progression in NAFLD [169] and is positively correlated with disease severity in NASH [24]. The failure of UPR in mitigating the ER stress leads to cell death via several mechanisms (**Figure 4**).

CHOP is one of the best characterized UPR-regulated pro-apoptotic protein [120]. CHOP is an ER-derived transcription factor activated downstream from PKR- and ATF6-pathway of UPR. Significance of CHOP in inducing apoptosis can be emphasized from results of study where silencing CHOP lead to decreased hepatocyte apoptosis in alcohol-induced liver disease [130] and attenuated cholestasis-induced liver fibrosis [170]. However, the role of CHOP is paradoxical in NAFLD, as demonstrated in study where CHOP deletion can reduce palmitate-induced apoptosis in hepatocyte cell line, whereas MCD diet-induced apoptosis was not reduced in CHOP knockout mice [171, 172].

CHOP has been described as an unstable protein compared to other protein chaperons like GRP78 [120]. Above described paradoxical role of CHOP in NAFLD makes way for observation: role of CHOP as a pro-apoptotic protein may be dependent on level of CHOP expression, the presence of factors which increase stability and/or protein–protein interactions that direct cell specific effects [173, 174]. Hence, future studies regarding role of CHOP in mice model are needed to elicit exact contributions of CHOP towards disease progression in NAFLD and NASH.

Furthermore, The IRE1 branch of the UPR, via its activation of JNK and Caspase 12 [175], and its interaction with Bax and Bak (two pro-apoptotic Bcl2 family members) [176], can also activate path towards apoptosis.

Additionally, another mechanism proposed for hepatic cell apoptosis is dysregulation in ER calcium flux. The ER calcium flux is regulated by ER stress, ER-localized protein and BCL-2 proteins interacting with other ER-localized proteins [177, 178]. The ERO1α-mediated activation of $IP_{3,}$ as mentioned earlier, can lead to disruption of ER calcium homeostasis [132]. This disruption inhibits sarco-endoplasmic reticulum Ca^{2+}-ATPase uptake pump, decreasing the folding capacity of ER, and hence, can induce ER stress and apoptosis [179]. Truncated variants of sarco-endoplasmic reticulum Ca^{2+}-ATPase have also been implicated in dysregulation

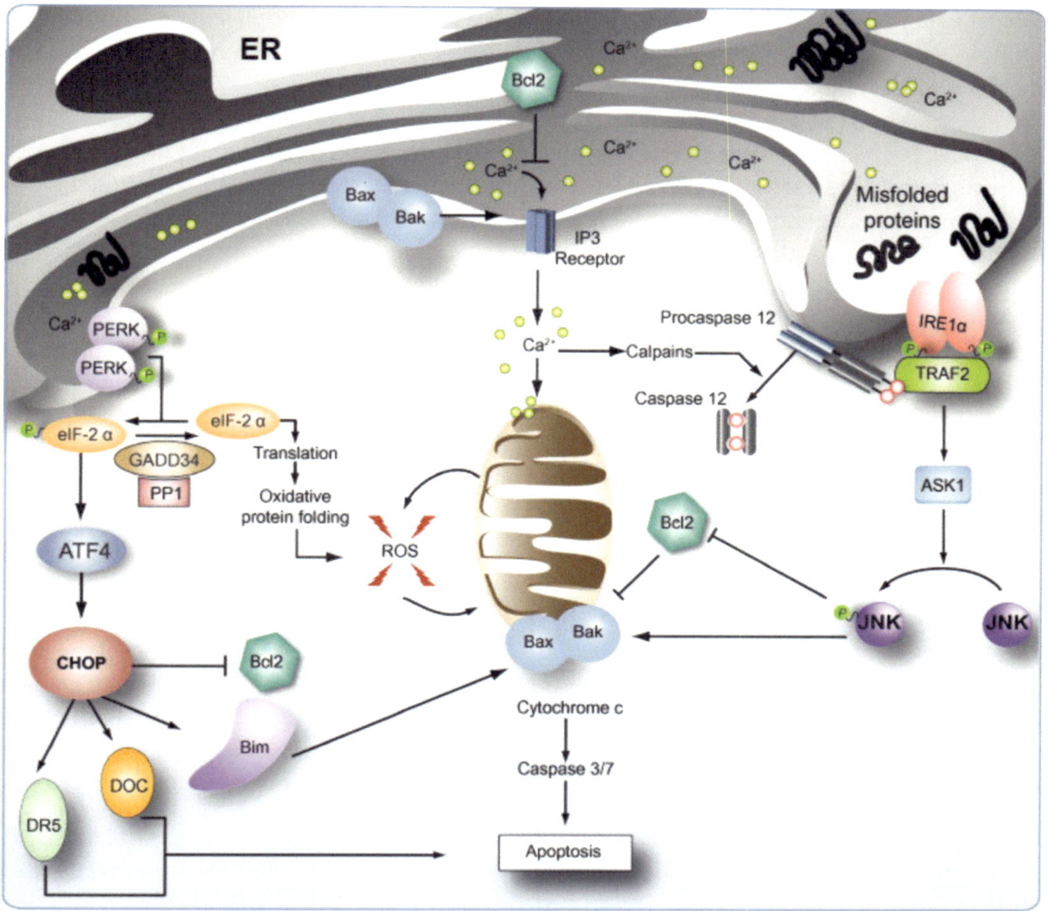

Figure 4. Different mechanisms for ER stress-induced apoptosis [135] (https://doi.org/10.1016/j.jhep.2010.11.005) (http://creativecommons.org/licenses/by-nc-nd/4.0/).

of Calcium flux [180]. Subsequently, the release of ER calcium and its uptake in mitochondria leads to mitochondrial membrane permeabilization, and activation of intrinsic apoptotic pathway. Recent studies also suggest that Smooth and Rough ER may be physically and functionally interacting with mitochondria via tethers and reduction in lengths of these tethers in response to pro-apoptotic agents might be one mechanism for apoptosis [181, 182].

7. Genetic factors

A possible explanation for observed inter-individual variability in susceptibility to NAFLD and progressive NASH is provided by genetics. *Patatin-like phospholipase domain-containing*

3 (PNPLA3), also called adiponutrin, is a protein expressed on endoplasmic reticulum, and on lipid droplets in hepatocytes and adipocytes [183]. It is activated after feeding and is the master regulator of lipogenesis by SREBP-1c. The 148 M variant of PNPLA3 is associated with increased expression of lipogenic transcription factor SREBP1c and alters the lipid catabolism [184]. The 148 M variant is associated with increased severity of NAFLD. In another study, patients with 148 M variant in genotype developed increased steatosis, with augmented lobular inflammation, hepatocellular ballooning and NASH [185].

7.1. Epigenetic modifications

Epigenetic modifications, mainly including microRNA, DNA methylation, histone modification and ubiquination, refers to phenotypic changes irrespective of changes to underlying DNA. "miRNA" are small single stranded RNA molecules regulating mRNA degradation or translation inhibition, subsequently altering protein expression of target genes [186]. The miR-122, which accounts for 70% of all miRNA in the liver, is significantly under-expressed in NASH subjects compared to normal subjects [187]. Inhibition of miR-122 via antisense oligonucleotide in diet-induced obesity mouse models resulted in decreased mRNA expression of acetyl-CoA carboxylase-2, fatty acid synthase, SREBP1c, Stearoyl-CoA desaturase, all of which are key lipogenic factors in human NASH, and the histology showed marked improvement in liver steatosis [188]. In another study in mice, the plasma cholesterol level, hepatic fatty acid and cholesterol synthesis rate as well as HMG CoA reductase level were all significantly reduced after silencing miR-122 [189]. These findings strongly suggest the significance miR-122 in the regulation of lipid metabolism. Besides miR-122, miR-34a and miR-146b were shown to be significantly over-expressed in human NASH [187].

Similarly, aberrant methylation patterns of genomic DNA have been linked to NAFLD. A recent study found positive correlation between NAFLD and hepatic DNA methylation of GpC in PPAR-δ and mitochondrial transcription factor A (TFAM), with methylation being higher in NAFLD liver as compared to control [190]. In conclusion, genetic and epigenetic factors interact with other determinants to produce NAFLD phenotype and determine the rate of its progression [187].

8. Conclusion

The above laborious and detailed discussion on complex molecular mechanisms associated with disease progression in NAFLD does point towards the fact: The pathogenesis and progression of disease in NAFLD is complex interplay of different hormonal, immunological, metabolic, genetic and environmental components. Each component can act on its own or act in concert with other culprits to causes augmented damage to liver. However, more studies are needed to uncover the still unknown players, and to understand the interactions between the different players of multiple-hit model.

http://dx.doi.org/10.5772/intechopen.71405

Appendix

ACC	acetyl-CoA carboxylase
AhR	aryl hydrocarbon receptor
AMPK	cyclin AMP dependent protein kinase
AP-1	activating protein-1
ASK1	apoptotic signal kinase-1
ATF6	activating transcription factor 6
CDAA diet	choline-deficient, amino acid defined diet
CHOP	CCAAT-enhancer-binding protein homologous protein
ChREBP	carbohydrate response element-binding protein
CREB	cAMP response element-binding protein
DAMP	danger associated molecular pattern
DGAT	diacylglycerol transferase
DR5	death receptor 5
eIF-2α	eukaryotic initiation factor-2α
ER	endoplasmic reticulum
Ero 1 α	endoplasmic reticulum oxidoreductase 1
Fiaf	fasting-induced adipocyte factor
FXR	farnesoid X receptor
GADD	growth arrest and DNA damage
HNE	4-hydroxy-2-noneal
IKKb	Inhibitor of nuclear factor kappa-B kinase subunit beta
Insigs	insulin regulated proteins
IRE 1	inositol-requiring ER-to-nucleus signaling protein1
IRS	insulin receptor substrate
JNK	Jun N-terminal Kinase

LPS	lipopolysaccharide
MAP	mitogen-activated protein
MAPK	mitogen-activated protein kinase
mTOR	mechanistic target of rapamycin
NAFLD	nonalcoholic fatty liver disease
NALP	NACHT, LRR and PYD domains-containing protein 3
NF-κB	nuclear factor κ beta
NLR	nod-like receptor
NLRP	NLR family, pyrin domain-containing 3 inflammasomes
Nrf2	nuclear factor-erythroid-derived 2-related factor 2
PERK	protein kinase RNA- like endoplasmic reticulum kinase
PKC-γ	protein kinase C-gamma
PKR	RNA activated protein kinase
PNPLA3	patatin-like phospholipase domain-containing 3
PPAR	peroxisome proliferator activated receptor
ROS	reactive oxygen species
SCAP	SREBP-cleavage activating proteins
SCD1	stearoyl-CoA desaturase-1
SCFA	short chain fatty acid
SOCS	suppressor of cytokine signaling
SREBP	sterol regulatory element-binding protein
TBARS	thiobarbituric acid reacting substrate
TFAM	mitochondrial transcription factor A
TGF-β1	transforming growth factor-β1
TLR	toll-like receptor
TNF	tumor necrosis factor

TNFR	tumor necrosis factor receptor
TRAIL	TNF-related apoptosis-inducing ligand
UPR	unfolded protein response
XBP1	X-box binding protein-1

Author details

Om Parkash[1]* and Subha Saeed[2]

*Address all correspondence to: om.parkash@aku.edu

1 Section of Gastroenterology/Hepatology, Department of Medicine, The Aga Khan University Hospital, Pakistan

2 The Aga Khan University Hospital, Pakistan

References

[1] AS Y, Keeffe EB. Nonalcoholic fatty liver disease. Reviews in Gastroenterological Disorders. 2002;**2**(1):11-19

[2] Vernon G, Baranova A, Younossi ZM. Systematic review: The epidemiology and natural history of non-alcoholic fatty liver disease and non-alcoholic steatohepatitis in adults. Alimentary Pharmacology & Therapeutics. 2011;**34**(3):274-285

[3] de Alwis NM, Day CP. Non-alcoholic fatty liver disease: The mist gradually clears. Journal of Hepatology. 2008;**48**(Suppl 1):S104-S112

[4] Law K, Brunt EM. Nonalcoholic fatty liver disease. Clinics in Liver Disease. 2010;**14**(4): 591-604

[5] Ekstedt M, Franzen LE, Mathiesen UL, Thorelius L, Holmqvist M, Bodemar G, et al. Long-term follow-up of patients with NAFLD and elevated liver enzymes. Hepatology (Baltimore, Md). 2006;**44**(4):865, 73

[6] Teli MR, James OF, Burt AD, Bennett MK, Day CP. The natural history of nonalcoholic fatty liver: A follow-up study. Hepatology (Baltimore, Md). 1995;**22**(6):1714, 9

[7] Day CP, James OF. Steatohepatitis: A tale of two "hits"? Gastroenterology. 1998;**114**(4): 842-845

[8] Buzzetti E, Pinzani M, Tsochatzis EA. The multiple-hit pathogenesis of non-alcoholic fatty liver disease (NAFLD). Metabolism, Clinical and Experimental. 2016;**65**(8):1038-1048

[9] Tilg H, Moschen AR. Evolution of inflammation in nonalcoholic fatty liver disease: The multiple parallel hits hypothesis. Hepatology (Baltimore, Md). 2010;**52**(5):1836-1846

[10] Fabbrini E, Mohammed BS, Magkos F, Korenblat KM, Patterson BW, Klein S. Alterations in adipose tissue and hepatic lipid kinetics in obese men and women with nonalcoholic fatty liver disease. Gastroenterology. 2008;**134**(2):424-431

[11] Donnelly KL, Smith CI, Schwarzenberg SJ, Jessurun J, Boldt MD, Parks EJ. Sources of fatty acids stored in liver and secreted via lipoproteins in patients with nonalcoholic fatty liver disease. The Journal of Clinical Investigation. 2005;**115**(5):1343-1351

[12] Schwarz JM, Linfoot P, Dare D, Aghajanian K. Hepatic de novo lipogenesis in normoinsulinemic and hyperinsulinemic subjects consuming high-fat, low-carbohydrate and low-fat, high-carbohydrate isoenergetic diets. The American Journal of Clinical Nutrition. 2003;**77**(1):43-50

[13] Lambert JE, Ramos-Roman MA, Browning JD, Parks EJ. Increased de novo lipogenesis is a distinct characteristic of individuals with nonalcoholic fatty liver disease. Gastroenterology. 2014;**146**(3):726-735

[14] Nehra V, Angulo P, Buchman AL, Lindor KD. Nutritional and metabolic considerations in the etiology of nonalcoholic steatohepatitis. Digestive Diseases and Sciences. 2001;**46**(11):2347-2352

[15] Malhi H, Gores GJ. Molecular mechanisms of lipotoxicity in nonalcoholic fatty liver disease. Seminars in Liver Disease. 2008;**28**(4):360-369

[16] Malhi H, Bronk SF, Werneburg NW, Gores GJ. Free fatty acids induce JNK-dependent hepatocyte lipoapoptosis. The Journal of Biological Chemistry. 2006;**281**(17):12093-12101

[17] Barreyro FJ, Kobayashi S, Bronk SF, Werneburg NW, Malhi H, Gores GJ. Transcriptional regulation of Bim by FoxO3A mediates hepatocyte lipoapoptosis. The Journal of Biological Chemistry. 2007;**282**(37):27141-27154

[18] Guicciardi ME, Leist M, Gores GJ. Lysosomes in cell death. Oncogene. 2004;**23**(16): 2881-2890

[19] Feldstein AE, Werneburg NW, Canbay A, Guicciardi ME, Bronk SF, Rydzewski R, et al. Free fatty acids promote hepatic lipotoxicity by stimulating TNF-alpha expression via a lysosomal pathway. Hepatology (Baltimore, Md). 2004;**40**(1):185-194

[20] Wei Y, Wang D, Topczewski F, Pagliassotti MJ. Saturated fatty acids induce endoplasmic reticulum stress and apoptosis independently of ceramide in liver cells. American Journal of Physiology. Endocrinology and Metabolism. 2006;**291**(2):E275-E281

[21] Hirosumi J, Tuncman G, Chang L, Gorgun CZ, Uysal KT, Maeda K, et al. A central role for JNK in obesity and insulin resistance. Nature. 2002;**420**(6913):333-336

[22] Kim BJ, Ryu SW, Song BJ. JNK- and p38 kinase-mediated phosphorylation of Bax leads to its activation and mitochondrial translocation and to apoptosis of human hepatoma HepG2 cells. The Journal of Biological Chemistry. 2006;**281**(30):21256-21265

[23] Yamamoto T, Nakade Y, Yamauchi T, Kobayashi Y, Ishii N, Ohashi T, et al. Glucagon-like peptide-1 analogue prevents nonalcoholic steatohepatitis in non-obese mice. World Journal of Gastroenterology. 2016;**22**(8):2512-2523

[24] Feldstein AE, Canbay A, Angulo P, Taniai M, Burgart LJ, Lindor KD, et al. Hepatocyte apoptosis and fas expression are prominent features of human nonalcoholic steatohepatitis. Gastroenterology. 2003;**125**(2):437-443

[25] Weisberg SP, McCann D, Desai M, Rosenbaum M, Leibel RL, Ferrante AW Jr. Obesity is associated with macrophage accumulation in adipose tissue. The Journal of Clinical Investigation. 2003;**112**(12):1796-1808

[26] Hotamisligil GS, Arner P, Caro JF, Atkinson RL, Spiegelman BM. Increased adipose tissue expression of tumor necrosis factor-alpha in human obesity and insulin resistance. The Journal of Clinical Investigation. 1995;**95**(5):2409-2415

[27] Feldstein AE, Canbay A, Guicciardi ME, Higuchi H, Bronk SF, Gores GJ. Diet associated hepatic steatosis sensitizes to Fas mediated liver injury in mice. Journal of Hepatology. 2003;**39**(6):978-983

[28] Mari M, Fernandez-Checa JC. Sphingolipid signalling and liver diseases. Liver international : official journal of the International Association for the Study of the Liver. 2007;**27**(4):440-450

[29] Paumen MB, Ishida Y, Muramatsu M, Yamamoto M, Honjo T. Inhibition of carnitine palmitoyltransferase I augments sphingolipid synthesis and palmitate-induced apoptosis. The Journal of Biological Chemistry. 1997;**272**(6):3324-3329

[30] Suganami T, Nishida J, Ogawa Y. A paracrine loop between adipocytes and macrophages aggravates inflammatory changes: Role of free fatty acids and tumor necrosis factor alpha. Arteriosclerosis, Thrombosis, and Vascular Biology. 2005;**25**(10):2062-2068

[31] Shi H, Kokoeva MV, Inouye K, Tzameli I, Yin H, Flier JS. TLR4 links innate immunity and fatty acid-induced insulin resistance. The Journal of Clinical Investigation. 2006;**116**(11):3015-3025

[32] Chalasani N, Deeg MA, Crabb DW. Systemic levels of lipid peroxidation and its metabolic and dietary correlates in patients with nonalcoholic steatohepatitis. The American Journal of Gastroenterology. 2004;**99**(8):1497-1502

[33] Seki S, Kitada T, Sakaguchi H. Clinicopathological significance of oxidative cellular damage in non-alcoholic fatty liver diseases. Hepatology Research: The Official Journal of the Japan Society of Hepatology. 2005;**33**(2):132-134

[34] Yesilova Z, Yaman H, Oktenli C, Ozcan A, Uygun A, Cakir E, et al. Systemic markers of lipid peroxidation and antioxidants in patients with nonalcoholic fatty liver disease. The American Journal of Gastroenterology. 2005;**100**(4):850-855

[35] Valenzuela R, Videla LA. The importance of the long-chain polyunsaturated fatty acid n-6/n-3 ratio in development of non-alcoholic fatty liver associated with obesity. Food & Function. 2011;**2**(11):644-648

[36] Lombardo YB, Chicco AG. Effects of dietary polyunsaturated n-3 fatty acids on dyslipidemia and insulin resistance in rodents and humans. A review. The Journal of Nutritional Biochemistry. 2006;**17**(1):1-13

[37] Valenzuela R, Barrera C, Espinosa A, Llanos P, Orellana P, Videla LA. Reduction in the desaturation capacity of the liver in mice subjected to high fat diet: Relation to LCPUFA depletion in liver and extrahepatic tissues. Prostaglandins, Leukotrienes and Essential Fatty Acids (PLEFA). 2015;**98**:7-14

[38] Puri P, Baillie RA, Wiest MM, Mirshahi F, Choudhury J, Cheung O, et al. A lipidomic analysis of nonalcoholic fatty liver disease. Hepatology (Baltimore, Md). 2007;**46**(4):1081-1090

[39] Mari M, Caballero F, Colell A, Morales A, Caballeria J, Fernandez A, et al. Mitochondrial free cholesterol loading sensitizes to TNF- and Fas-mediated steatohepatitis. Cell Metabolism. 2006;**4**(3):185-198

[40] Koliwad SK, Streeper RS, Monetti M, Cornelissen I, Chan L, Terayama K, et al. DGAT1-dependent triacylglycerol storage by macrophages protects mice from diet-induced insulin resistance and inflammation. The Journal of Clinical Investigation. 2010;**120**(3):756-767

[41] Yamaguchi K, Yang L, McCall S, Huang J, Yu XX, Pandey SK, et al. Inhibiting triglyceride synthesis improves hepatic steatosis but exacerbates liver damage and fibrosis in obese mice with nonalcoholic steatohepatitis. Hepatology (Baltimore, Md). 2007;**45**(6): 1366-1374

[42] Unger RH, Scherer PE. Gluttony, sloth and the metabolic syndrome: A roadmap to lipotoxicity. Trends in Endocrinology and Metabolism: TEM. 2010;**21**(6):345-352

[43] Lin HZ, Yang SQ, Chuckaree C, Kuhajda F, Ronnet G, Diehl AM. Metformin reverses fatty liver disease in obese, leptin-deficient mice. Nature Medicine. 2000;**6**(9):998-1003

[44] Li Z, Yang S, Lin H, Huang J, Watkins PA, Moser AB, et al. Probiotics and antibodies to TNF inhibit inflammatory activity and improve nonalcoholic fatty liver disease. Hepatology (Baltimore, Md). 2003;**37**(2):343-350

[45] Tilg H, Jalan R, Kaser A, Davies NA, Offner FA, Hodges SJ, et al. Anti-tumor necrosis factor-alpha monoclonal antibody therapy in severe alcoholic hepatitis. Journal of Hepatology. 2003;**38**(4):419-425

[46] Clementi AH, Gaudy AM, van Rooijen N, Pierce RH, Mooney RA. Loss of Kupffer cells in diet-induced obesity is associated with increased hepatic steatosis, STAT3

signaling, and further decreases in insulin signaling. Biochimica et Biophysica Acta. 2009; **1792**(11):1062-1072

[47] Bugianesi E, Gastaldelli A, Vanni E, Gambino R, Cassader M, Baldi S, et al. Insulin resistance in non-diabetic patients with non-alcoholic fatty liver disease: Sites and mechanisms. Diabetologia. 2005;**48**(4):634-642

[48] Sabio G, Das M, Mora A, Zhang Z, Jun JY, Ko HJ, et al. A stress signaling pathway in adipose tissue regulates hepatic insulin resistance. Science (New York, N.Y.). 2008; **322**(5907):1539-1543

[49] Taniguchi CM, Emanuelli B, Kahn CR. Critical nodes in signalling pathways: Insights into insulin action. Nature Reviews. Molecular Cell Biology. 2006;**7**(2):85-96

[50] Luyckx F, Lefebvre P, Scheen A. Non-alcoholic steatohepatitis: Association with obesity and insulin resistance, and influence of weight loss. Diabetes & Metabolism. 2000; **26**(2):98-106

[51] Lam TK, Carpentier A, Lewis GF, van de Werve G, Fantus IG, Giacca A. Mechanisms of the free fatty acid-induced increase in hepatic glucose production. American Journal of Physiology-Endocrinology and Metabolism. 2003;**284**(5):E863-EE73

[52] Videla LA, Rodrigo R, Araya J, Poniachik J. Insulin resistance and oxidative stress interdependency in non-alcoholic fatty liver disease. Trends in Molecular Medicine. 2006; **12**(12):555-558

[53] Houstis N, Rosen E, Lander E. Reactive oxygen species have a causal role in multiple forms of insulin resistance. Nature. 2006;**440**:944-948. Find this article online

[54] Woodcroft KJ, Hafner MS, Novak RF. Insulin signaling in the transcriptional and post-transcriptional regulation of CYP2E1 expression. Hepatology. 2002;**35**(2):263-273

[55] Stefan N, Kantartzis K, Häring H-U. Causes and metabolic consequences of fatty liver. Endocrine Reviews. 2008;**29**(7):939-960

[56] Peverill W, Powell LW, Skoien R. Evolving concepts in the pathogenesis of NASH: Beyond steatosis and inflammation. International Journal of Molecular Sciences. 2014; **15**(5):8591-8638

[57] Arumugam M, Raes J, Pelletier E, Le Paslier D, Yamada T, Mende DR, et al. Enterotypes of the human gut microbiome. Nature. 2011;**473**(7346):174-180

[58] Turnbaugh PJ, Ley RE, Mahowald MA, Magrini V, Mardis ER, Gordon JI. An obesity-associated gut microbiome with increased capacity for energy harvest. Nature. 2006; **444**(7122):1027-1131

[59] Miele L, Valenza V, La Torre G, Montalto M, Cammarota G, Ricci R, et al. Increased intestinal permeability and tight junction alterations in nonalcoholic fatty liver disease. Hepatology (Baltimore, Md). 2009;**49**(6):1877-1887

[60] Brun P, Castagliuolo I, Di Leo V, Buda A, Pinzani M, Palù G, et al. Increased intestinal permeability in obese mice: New evidence in the pathogenesis of nonalcoholic steatohepatitis. American Journal of Physiology. Gastrointestinal and Liver Physiology. 2007;**292**(2):G518-GG25

[61] Cani PD, Bibiloni R, Knauf C, Waget A, Neyrinck AM, Delzenne NM, et al. Changes in gut microbiota control metabolic endotoxemia-induced inflammation in high-fat diet-induced obesity and diabetes in mice. Diabetes. 2008;**57**(6):1470-1481

[62] Cani PD, Amar J, Iglesias MA, Poggi M, Knauf C, Bastelica D, et al. Metabolic endotoxemia initiates obesity and insulin resistance. Diabetes. 2007;**56**(7):1761-1772

[63] Noverr MC, Huffnagle GB. Does the microbiota regulate immune responses outside the gut? Trends in Microbiology. 2004;**12**(12):562-568

[64] Rivera CA, Adegboyega P, van Rooijen N, Tagalicud A, Allman M, Wallace M. Toll-like receptor-4 signaling and Kupffer cells play pivotal roles in the pathogenesis of non-alcoholic steatohepatitis. Journal of Hepatology. 2007;**47**(4):571-579

[65] Pappo I, Becovier H, Berry EM, Freund HR. Polymyxin B reduces cecal flora, TNF production and hepatic steatosis during total parenteral nutrition in the rat. The Journal of Surgical Research. 1991;**51**(2):106-112

[66] Topping DL, Clifton PM. Short-chain fatty acids and human colonic function: Roles of resistant starch and nonstarch polysaccharides. Physiological Reviews. 2001; **81**(3):1031-1064

[67] Vernia P, Marcheggiano A, Caprilli R, Frieri G, Corrao G, Valpiani D, et al. Short-chain fatty acid topical treatment in distal ulcerative colitis. Alimentary Pharmacology & Therapeutics. 1995;**9**(3):309-313

[68] Maslowski KM, Vieira AT, Ng A, Kranich J, Sierro F, Yu D, et al. Regulation of inflammatory responses by gut microbiota and chemoattractant receptor GPR43. Nature. 2009;**461**(7268):1282-1286

[69] Zeisel SH, Wishnok JS, Blusztajn J. Formation of methylamines from ingested choline and lecithin. The Journal of Pharmacology and Experimental Therapeutics. 1983; **225**(2):320-324

[70] Abu-Shanab A, Quigley EM. The role of the gut microbiota in nonalcoholic fatty liver disease. Nature Reviews Gastroenterology & Hepatology. 2010;**7**(12):691-701

[71] Zhu L, Baker SS, Gill C, Liu W, Alkhouri R, Baker RD, et al. Characterization of gut microbiomes in nonalcoholic steatohepatitis (NASH) patients: A connection between endogenous alcohol and NASH. Hepatology (Baltimore, Md). 2013;**57**(2):601-609

[72] Lieber CS. Role of S-adenosyl-L-methionine in the treatment of liver diseases. Journal of Hepatology. 1999;**30**(6):1155-1159

[73] Henao-Mejia J, Elinav E, Jin C, Hao L, Mehal WZ, Strowig T, et al. Inflammasome-mediated dysbiosis regulates progression of NAFLD and obesity. Nature. 2012;**482**(7384):179-185

[74] Tremaroli V, Bäckhed F. Functional interactions between the gut microbiota and host metabolism. Nature. 2012;**489**(7415):242-249

[75] Sinal CJ, Tohkin M, Miyata M, Ward JM, Lambert G, Gonzalez FJ. Targeted disruption of the nuclear receptor FXR/BAR impairs bile acid and lipid homeostasis. Cell. 2000;**102**(6):731-744

[76] Cariou B. The farnesoid X receptor (FXR) as a new target in non-alcoholic steatohepatitis. Diabetes & Metabolism. 2008;**34**(6):685-691

[77] Tetri LH, Basaranoglu M, Brunt EM, Yerian LM, Neuschwander-Tetri BA. Severe NAFLD with hepatic necroinflammatory changes in mice fed trans fats and a high-fructose corn syrup equivalent. American Journal of Physiology. Gastrointestinal and Liver Physiology. 2008;**295**(5):G987-G995

[78] Bergheim I, Weber S, Vos M, Krämer S, Volynets V, Kaserouni S, et al. Antibiotics protect against fructose-induced hepatic lipid accumulation in mice: Role of endotoxin. Journal of Hepatology. 2008;**48**(6):983-992

[79] Abdelmalek MF, Suzuki A, Guy C, Unalp-Arida A, Colvin R, Johnson RJ, et al. Increased fructose consumption is associated with fibrosis severity in patients with nonalcoholic fatty liver disease. Hepatology. 2010;**51**(6):1961-1971

[80] Lim JS, Mietus-Snyder M, Valente A, Schwarz J-M, Lustig RH. The role of fructose in the pathogenesis of NAFLD and the metabolic syndrome. Nature Reviews. Gastroenterology & Hepatology. 2010;**7**(5):251-264

[81] Lanaspa MA, Sanchez-Lozada LG, Choi Y-J, Cicerchi C, Kanbay M, Roncal-Jimenez CA, et al. Uric acid induces hepatic steatosis by generation of mitochondrial oxidative stress potential role in fructose-dependent and-independent fatty liver. The Journal of Biological Chemistry. 2012;**287**(48):40732-40744

[82] Pérez-Carreras M, Del Hoyo P, Martín MA, Rubio JC, Martín A, Castellano G, et al. Defective hepatic mitochondrial respiratory chain in patients with nonalcoholic steatohepatitis. Hepatology. 2003;**38**(4):999-1007

[83] Jegatheesan P, De Bandt JP. Fructose and NAFLD: The multifaceted aspects of fructose metabolism. Nutrients. 2017;**9**(3):230

[84] Stevens EA, Mezrich JD, Bradfield CA. The aryl hydrocarbon receptor: A perspective on potential roles in the immune system. Immunology. 2009;**127**(3):299-311

[85] Lee JH, Wada T, Febbraio M, He J, Matsubara T, Lee MJ, et al. A novel role for the dioxin receptor in fatty acid metabolism and hepatic steatosis. Gastroenterology. 2010;**139**(2):653-663

[86] Hernandez-Rodas MC, Valenzuela R, Videla LA. Relevant aspects of nutritional and dietary interventions in non-alcoholic fatty liver disease. International Journal of Molecular Sciences. 2015;**16**(10):25168-25198

[87] Xu A. The fat-derived hormone adiponectin alleviates alcoholic and nonalcoholic fatty liver diseases in mice. Journal of Clinical Investigation. 2003;**112**(1):91-100

[88] Arita Y, Kihara S, Ouchi N, Takahashi M, Maeda K, Miyagawa J, et al. Paradoxical decrease of an adipose-specific protein, adiponectin, in obesity. Biochemical and Biophysical Research Communications. 1999;**257**(1):79-83

[89] Weyer C, Funahashi T, Tanaka S, Hotta K, Matsuzawa Y, Pratley RE, et al. Hypoadiponectinemia in obesity and type 2 diabetes: Close association with insulin resistance and hyperinsulinemia. The Journal of Clinical Endocrinology and Metabolism. 2001;**86**(5):1930-1935

[90] Takaki A, Kawai D, Yamamoto K. Multiple hits, including oxidative stress, as pathogenesis and treatment target in non-alcoholic steatohepatitis (NASH). International Journal of Molecular Sciences. 2013;**14**(10):20704-20728

[91] Kaser S, Moschen A, Cayon A, Kaser A, Crespo J, Pons-Romero F, et al. Adiponectin and its receptors in non-alcoholic steatohepatitis. Gut. 2005;**54**(1):117-121

[92] Yamauchi T, Kamon J, Minokoshi YA, Ito Y, Waki H, Uchida S, et al. Adiponectin stimulates glucose utilization and fatty-acid oxidation by activating AMP-activated protein kinase. Nature Medicine. 2002;**8**(11):1288-1295

[93] Tilg H, Moschen AR. Adipocytokines: Mediators linking adipose tissue, inflammation and immunity. Nature Reviews Immunology. 2006;**6**(10):772-783

[94] Yamauchi T, Kamon J, Ito Y, Tsuchida A, Yokomizo T, Kita S, et al. Cloning of adiponectin receptors that mediate antidiabetic metabolic effects. Nature. 2003;**423**(6941):762-769

[95] Maeda N, Takahashi M, Funahashi T, Kihara S, Nishizawa H, Kishida K, et al. PPARγ ligands increase expression and plasma concentrations of adiponectin, an adipose-derived protein. Diabetes. 2001;**50**(9):2094-2099

[96] Friedman JM, Leibel R, Siegel D, Walsh J, Bahary N. Molecular mapping of the mouse ob mutation. Genomics. 1991;**11**(4):1054-1062

[97] Carbone F, La Rocca C, Matarese G. Immunological functions of leptin and adiponectin. Biochimie. 2012;**94**(10):2082-2088

[98] Polyzos SA, Kountouras J, Mantzoros CS. Leptin in nonalcoholic fatty liver disease: A narrative review. Metabolism, Clinical and Experimental. 2015;**64**(1):60-78

[99] Choi SS, Syn W-K, Karaca GF, Omenetti A, Moylan CA, Witek RP, et al. Leptin promotes the myofibroblastic phenotype in hepatic stellate cells by activating the hedgehog pathway. The Journal of Biological Chemistry. 2010;**285**(47):36551-36560

[100] Aleffi S, Navari N, Delogu W, Galastri S, Novo E, Rombouts K, et al. Mammalian target of rapamycin mediates the angiogenic effects of leptin in human hepatic stellate cells. American Journal of Physiology. Gastrointestinal and Liver Physiology. 2011;**301**(2):G210-G2G9

[101] Wang J, Leclercq I, Brymora JM, Xu N, Ramezani-Moghadam M, London RM, et al. Kupffer cells mediate leptin-induced liver fibrosis. Gastroenterology. 2009;**137**(2):713-723. e1

[102] Imajo K, Fujita K, Yoneda M, Nozaki Y, Ogawa Y, Shinohara Y, et al. Hyperresponsivity to low-dose endotoxin during progression to nonalcoholic steatohepatitis is regulated by leptin-mediated signaling. Cell Metabolism. 2012;**16**(1):44-54

[103] Polyzos SA, Aronis KN, Kountouras J, Raptis DD, Vasiloglou MF, Mantzoros CS. Circulating Leptin in Non-alcoholic Fatty Liver Disease: A Systematic Review and Meta-Analysis. Springer; 2016

[104] Poniachik J, Csendes A, Díaz JC, Rojas J, Burdiles P, Maluenda F, Videla LA. Increased production of IL-1α and TNF-α in lipopolysaccharide-stimulated blood from obese patients with non-alcoholic fatty liver disease. Santiago, Chile: Cytokine; 2006;**33**(5):252-257

[105] Hotamisligil GS, Shargill NS, Spiegelman BM. Adipose expression of tumor necrosis factor-alpha: Direct role in obesity-linked insulin resistance. Science (New York, N.Y.). 1993;**259**(5091):87-91

[106] Fernandez-Real JM, Vayreda M, Richart C, Gutierrez C, Broch M, Vendrell J, et al. Circulating interleukin 6 levels, blood pressure, and insulin sensitivity in apparently healthy men and women. The Journal of Clinical Endocrinology and Metabolism. 2001;**86**(3):1154-1159

[107] Tomita K, Tamiya G, Ando S, Ohsumi K, Chiyo T, Mizutani A, et al. Tumour necrosis factor α signalling through activation of Kupffer cells plays an essential role in liver fibrosis of non-alcoholic steatohepatitis in mice. Gut. 2006;**55**(3):415-424

[108] Senn JJ, Klover PJ, Nowak IA, Zimmers TA, Koniaris LG, Furlanetto RW, et al. Suppressor of cytokine signaling-3 (SOCS-3), a potential mediator of interleukin-6-dependent insulin resistance in hepatocytes. The Journal of Biological Chemistry. 2003;**278**(16):13740-13746

[109] Cai D, Yuan M, Frantz DF, Melendez PA, Hansen L, Lee J, et al. Local and systemic insulin resistance resulting from hepatic activation of IKK-β and NF-κB. Nature Medicine. 2005;**11**(2):183-190

[110] Ribeiro PS, Cortez-Pinto H, Solá S, Castro RE, Ramalho RM, Baptista A, et al. Hepatocyte apoptosis, expression of death receptors, and activation of NF-κB in the liver of nonalcoholic and alcoholic steatohepatitis patients. The American Journal of Gastroenterology. 2004;**99**(9):1708-1717

[111] Yu HB, Finlay BB. The caspase-1 inflammasome: A pilot of innate immune responses. Cell Host & Microbe. 2008;**4**(3):198-208

[112] Csak T, Ganz M, Pespisa J, Kodys K, Dolganiuc A, Szabo G. Fatty acid and endotoxin activate inflammasomes in mouse hepatocytes that release danger signals to stimulate immune cells. Hepatology (Baltimore, Md). 2011;**54**(1):133-144

[113] Wree A, McGeough MD, Peña CA, Schlattjan M, Li H, Inzaugarat ME, et al. NLRP3 inflammasome activation is required for fibrosis development in NAFLD. Journal of Molecular Medicine. 2014;**92**(10):1069-1082

[114] Miura K, Kodama Y, Inokuchi S, Schnabl B, Aoyama T, Ohnishi H, et al. Toll-like receptor 9 promotes steatohepatitis by induction of interleukin-1beta in mice. Gastroenterology. 2010;**139**(1):323-334. e7

[115] Nagy LE. Recent insights into the role of the innate immune system in the development of alcoholic liver disease. Experimental Biology and Medicine. 2003;**228**(8):882-890

[116] Spruss A, Kanuri G, Wagnerberger S, Haub S, Bischoff SC, Bergheim I. Toll-like receptor 4 is involved in the development of fructose-induced hepatic steatosis in mice. Hepatology (Baltimore, Md). 2009;**50**(4):1094-1104

[117] Miura K, Yang L, van Rooijen N, Brenner DA, Ohnishi H, Seki E. Toll-like receptor 2 and palmitic acid cooperatively contribute to the development of nonalcoholic steatohepatitis through inflammasome activation in mice. Hepatology (Baltimore, Md). 2013;**57**(2):577-589

[118] Vijay-Kumar M, Aitken JD, Carvalho FA, Cullender TC, Mwangi S, Srinivasan S, et al. Metabolic syndrome and altered gut microbiota in mice lacking toll-like receptor 5. Science (New York, N.Y.). 2010;**328**(5975):228-231

[119] Letran SE, Lee S-J, Atif SM, Flores-Langarica A, Uematsu S, Akira S, et al. TLR5-deficient mice lack basal inflammatory and metabolic defects but exhibit impaired CD4 T cell responses to a flagellated pathogen. The Journal of Immunology. 2011;**186**(9):5406-5412

[120] Gentile CL, Frye M, Pagliassotti MJ. Endoplasmic reticulum stress and the unfolded protein response in nonalcoholic fatty liver disease. Antioxidants & Redox Signaling. 2011;**15**(2):505-521

[121] Ashraf NU, Sheikh TA. Endoplasmic reticulum stress and oxidative stress in the pathogenesis of non-alcoholic fatty liver disease. Free Radical Research. 2015;**49**(12):1405-1418

[122] Schroder M, Kaufman RJ. ER stress and the unfolded protein response. Mutation Research. 2005;**569**(1-2):29-63

[123] Ozcan U, Cao Q, Yilmaz E, Lee AH, Iwakoshi NN, Ozdelen E, et al. Endoplasmic reticulum stress links obesity, insulin action, and type 2 diabetes. Science (New York, N.Y.). 2004;**306**(5695):457-461

[124] Wu J, Kaufman RJ. From acute ER stress to physiological roles of the unfolded protein response. Cell Death and Differentiation. 2006;**13**(3):374-384

[125] Zhang K, Kaufman RJ. From endoplasmic-reticulum stress to the inflammatory response. Nature. 2008;**454**(7203):455-462

[126] Ron D, Walter P. Signal integration in the endoplasmic reticulum unfolded protein response. Nature Reviews. Molecular Cell Biology. 2007;**8**(7):519-529

[127] Sano R, Reed JCER. Stress-induced cell death mechanisms. Biochimica et Biophysica Acta. 2013;**1833**(12):3460-3470

[128] Sozen E, Ozer NK. Impact of high cholesterol and endoplasmic reticulum stress on metabolic diseases: An updated mini-review. Redox Biology. 2017;**12**:456-461

[129] Harding HP, Zhang Y, Zeng H, Novoa I, Lu PD, Calfon M, et al. An integrated stress response regulates amino acid metabolism and resistance to oxidative stress. Molecular Cell. 2003;**11**(3):619-633

[130] Ji C, Mehrian-Shai R, Chan C, Hsu YH, Kaplowitz N. Role of CHOP in hepatic apoptosis in the murine model of intragastric ethanol feeding. Alcoholism, Clinical and Experimental Research. 2005;**29**(8):1496-1503

[131] Novoa I, Zeng H, Harding HP, Ron D. Feedback inhibition of the unfolded protein response by GADD34-mediated dephosphorylation of eIF2alpha. The Journal of Cell Biology. 2001;**153**(5):1011-1022

[132] Li G, Mongillo M, Chin KT, Harding H, Ron D, Marks AR, et al. Role of ERO1-alpha-mediated stimulation of inositol 1,4,5-triphosphate receptor activity in endoplasmic reticulum stress-induced apoptosis. The Journal of Cell Biology. 2009;**186**(6):783-792

[133] McCullough KD, Martindale JL, Klotz LO, Aw TY, Holbrook NJ. Gadd153 sensitizes cells to endoplasmic reticulum stress by down-regulating Bcl2 and perturbing the cellular redox state. Molecular and Cellular Biology. 2001;**21**(4):1249-1259

[134] Wang XZ, Ron D. Stress-induced phosphorylation and activation of the transcription factor CHOP (GADD153) by p38 MAP kinase. Science (New York, N.Y.). 1996; **272**(5266):1347-1349

[135] Malhi H, Kaufman RJ. Endoplasmic reticulum stress in liver disease. Journal of Hepatology. 2011;**54**(4):795-809

[136] Hu P, Han Z, Couvillon AD, Kaufman RJ, Exton JH. Autocrine tumor necrosis factor alpha links endoplasmic reticulum stress to the membrane death receptor pathway through IRE1alpha-mediated NF-kappaB activation and down-regulation of TRAF2 expression. Molecular and Cellular Biology. 2006;**26**(8):3071-3084

[137] Ron D, Hubbard SR. How IRE1 reacts to ER stress. Cell. 2008;**132**(1):24-26

[138] Davis RJ. Signal transduction by the JNK group of MAP kinases. Cell. 2000;**103**(2):239-252

[139] Amemiya-Kudo M, Shimano H, Hasty AH, Yahagi N, Yoshikawa T, Matsuzaka T, et al. Transcriptional activities of nuclear SREBP-1a, −1c, and −2 to different target promoters of lipogenic and cholesterogenic genes. The Journal of Lipid Research. 2002; **43**(8):1220-1235

[140] Brown MS, Goldstein JL. The SREBP pathway: Regulation of cholesterol metabolism by proteolysis of a membrane-bound transcription factor. Cell. 1997;**89**(3):331-340

[141] Yang T, Espenshade PJ, Wright ME, Yabe D, Gong Y, Aebersold R, et al. Crucial step in cholesterol homeostasis: Sterols promote binding of SCAP to INSIG-1, a membrane protein that facilitates retention of SREBPs in ER. Cell. 2002;**110**(4):489-500

[142] Lee JN, Ye J. Proteolytic activation of sterol regulatory element-binding protein induced by cellular stress through depletion of Insig-1. The Journal of Biological Chemistry. 2004;**279**(43):45257-45265

[143] Kammoun HL, Chabanon H, Hainault I, Luquet S, Magnan C, Koike T, et al. GRP78 expression inhibits insulin and ER stress-induced SREBP-1c activation and reduces hepatic steatosis in mice. The Journal of Clinical Investigation. 2009;**119**(5):1201-1215

[144] Lee JS, Zheng Z, Mendez R, Ha SW, Xie Y, Zhang K. Pharmacologic ER stress induces non-alcoholic steatohepatitis in an animal model. Toxicology Letters. 2012;**211**(1):29-38

[145] Rutkowski DT, Wu J, Back SH, Callaghan MU, Ferris SP, Iqbal J, et al. UPR pathways combine to prevent hepatic steatosis caused by ER stress-mediated suppression of transcriptional master regulators. Developmental Cell. 2008;**15**(6):829-840

[146] Bobrovnikova-Marjon E, Hatzivassiliou G, Grigoriadou C, Romero M, Cavener DR, Thompson CB, et al. PERK-dependent regulation of lipogenesis during mouse mammary gland development and adipocyte differentiation. Proceedings of the National Academy of Sciences of the United States of America. 2008;**105**(42):16314-16319

[147] Oyadomari S, Harding HP, Zhang Y, Oyadomari M, Ron D. Dephosphorylation of translation initiation factor 2alpha enhances glucose tolerance and attenuates hepatosteatosis in mice. Cell Metabolism. 2008;**7**(6):520-532

[148] Seo J, Fortuno ES 3rd, Suh JM, Stenesen D, Tang W, Parks EJ, et al. Atf4 regulates obesity, glucose homeostasis, and energy expenditure. Diabetes. 2009;**58**(11):2565-2573

[149] Xiao G, Zhang T, Yu S, Lee S, Calabuig-Navarro V, Yamauchi J, et al. ATF4 protein deficiency protects against high fructose-induced hypertriglyceridemia in mice. The Journal of Biological Chemistry. 2013;**288**(35):25350-25361

[150] Wang S, Chen Z, Lam V, Han J, Hassler J, Finck BN, et al. IRE1alpha-XBP1s induces PDI expression to increase MTP activity for hepatic VLDL assembly and lipid homeostasis. Cell Metabolism. 2012;**16**(4):473-486

[151] Zhang K, Wang S, Malhotra J, Hassler JR, Back SH, Wang G, et al. The unfolded protein response transducer IRE1alpha prevents ER stress-induced hepatic steatosis. The EMBO Journal. 2011;**30**(7):1357-1375

[152] Lee AH, Scapa EF, Cohen DE, Glimcher LH. Regulation of hepatic lipogenesis by the transcription factor XBP1. Science (New York, N.Y.). 2008;**320**(5882):1492-1496

[153] Zeng L, Lu M, Mori K, Luo S, Lee AS, Zhu Y, et al. ATF6 modulates SREBP2-mediated lipogenesis. The EMBO Journal. 2004;**23**(4):950-958

[154] Yamamoto K, Takahara K, Oyadomari S, Okada T, Sato T, Harada A, et al. Induction of liver steatosis and lipid droplet formation in ATF6alpha-knockout mice burdened with pharmacological endoplasmic reticulum stress. Molecular Biology of the Cell. 2010;**21**(17):2975-2986

[155] Santos CX, Tanaka LY, Wosniak J, Laurindo FR. Mechanisms and implications of reactive oxygen species generation during the unfolded protein response: Roles of endoplasmic reticulum oxidoreductases, mitochondrial electron transport, and NADPH oxidase. Antioxidants & Redox Signaling. 2009;**11**(10):2409-2427

[156] Hanada S, Harada M, Kumemura H, Bishr Omary M, Koga H, Kawaguchi T, et al. Oxidative stress induces the endoplasmic reticulum stress and facilitates inclusion formation in cultured cells. Journal of Hepatology. 2007;**47**(1):93-102

[157] Cullinan SB, Diehl JA. Coordination of ER and oxidative stress signaling: The PERK/Nrf2 signaling pathway. The International Journal of Biochemistry & Cell Biology. 2006;**38**(3):317-332

[158] Sugimoto H, Okada K, Shoda J, Warabi E, Ishige K, Ueda T, et al. Deletion of nuclear factor-E2-related factor-2 leads to rapid onset and progression of nutritional steatohepatitis in mice. American Journal of Physiology. Gastrointestinal and Liver Physiology. 2010;**298**(2):G283-G294

[159] Cullinan SB, Zhang D, Hannink M, Arvisais E, Kaufman RJ, Diehl JA. Nrf2 is a direct PERK substrate and effector of PERK-dependent cell survival. Molecular and Cellular Biology. 2003;**23**(20):7198-7209

[160] Liu Y, Adachi M, Zhao S, Hareyama M, Koong AC, Luo D, et al. Preventing oxidative stress: A new role for XBP1. Cell Death and Differentiation. 2009;**16**(6):847-857

[161] Urano F, Wang X, Bertolotti A, Zhang Y, Chung P, Harding HP, et al. Coupling of stress in the ER to activation of JNK protein kinases by transmembrane protein kinase IRE1. Science (New York, N.Y.). 2000;**287**(5453):664-666

[162] Jiang H-Y, Wek SA, McGrath BC, Scheuner D, Kaufman RJ, Cavener DR, et al. Phosphorylation of the α subunit of eukaryotic initiation factor 2 is required for activation of NF-κB in response to diverse cellular stresses. Molecular and Cellular Biology. 2003;**23**(16):5651-5663

[163] Yamazaki H, Hiramatsu N, Hayakawa K, Tagawa Y, Okamura M, Ogata R, et al. Activation of the Akt-NF-κB pathway by subtilase cytotoxin through the ATF6 branch of the unfolded protein response. The Journal of Immunology. 2009;**183**(2):1480-1487

[164] Donze O, Abbas-Terki T, Picard D. The Hsp90 chaperone complex is both a facilitator and a repressor of the dsRNA-dependent kinase PKR. The EMBO Journal. 2001;**20**(14):3771-3780

[165] Nakamura T, Furuhashi M, Li P, Cao H, Tuncman G, Sonenberg N, et al. Double-stranded RNA-dependent protein kinase links pathogen sensing with stress and metabolic homeostasis. Cell. 2010;**140**(3):338-348

[166] Donze O, Deng J, Curran J, Sladek R, Picard D, Sonenberg N. The protein kinase PKR: A molecular clock that sequentially activates survival and death programs. The EMBO Journal. 2004;**23**(3):564-571

[167] Luebke-Wheeler J, Zhang K, Battle M, Si-Tayeb K, Garrison W, Chhinder S, et al. Hepatocyte nuclear factor 4alpha is implicated in endoplasmic reticulum stress-induced acute phase response by regulating expression of cyclic adenosine monophosphate responsive element binding protein H. Hepatology (Baltimore, Md). 2008;**48**(4):1242-1250

[168] Zhang K, Shen X, Wu J, Sakaki K, Saunders T, Rutkowski DT, et al. Endoplasmic reticulum stress activates cleavage of CREBH to induce a systemic inflammatory response. Cell. 2006;**124**(3):587-599

[169] Wieckowska A, Zein NN, Yerian LM, Lopez AR, McCullough AJ, Feldstein AE. In vivo assessment of liver cell apoptosis as a novel biomarker of disease severity in nonalcoholic fatty liver disease. Hepatology (Baltimore, Md). 2006;**44**(1):27-33

[170] Tamaki N, Hatano E, Taura K, Tada M, Kodama Y, Nitta T, et al. CHOP deficiency attenuates cholestasis-induced liver fibrosis by reduction of hepatocyte injury. American Journal of Physiology. Gastrointestinal and Liver Physiology. 2008;**294**(2):G498-G505

[171] Pfaffenbach KT, Gentile CL, Nivala AM, Wang D, Wei Y, Pagliassotti MJ. Linking endoplasmic reticulum stress to cell death in hepatocytes: Roles of C/EBP homologous protein and chemical chaperones in palmitate-mediated cell death. American Journal of Physiology - Endocrinology and Metabolism. 2010;**298**(5):E1027-E1E35

[172] Zhang XQ, CF X, CH Y, Chen WX, Li YM. Role of endoplasmic reticulum stress in the pathogenesis of nonalcoholic fatty liver disease. World Journal of Gastroenterology. 2014;**20**(7):1768-1776

[173] Rutkowski DT, Arnold SM, Miller CN, Wu J, Li J, Gunnison KM, et al. Adaptation to ER stress is mediated by differential stabilities of pro-survival and pro-apoptotic mRNAs and proteins. PLoS Biology. 2006;**4**(11):e374

[174] Masciarelli S, Fra AM, Pengo N, Bertolotti M, Cenci S, Fagioli C, et al. CHOP-independent apoptosis and pathway-selective induction of the UPR in developing plasma cells. Molecular Immunology. 2010;**47**(6):1356-1365

[175] Yoneda T, Imaizumi K, Oono K, Yui D, Gomi F, Katayama T, et al. Activation of caspase-12, an endoplastic reticulum (ER) resident caspase, through tumor necrosis factor receptor-associated factor 2-dependent mechanism in response to the ER stress. The Journal of Biological Chemistry. 2001;**276**(17):13935-13940

[176] Hetz C, Bernasconi P, Fisher J, Lee A-H, Bassik MC, Antonsson B, et al. Proapoptotic BAX and BAK modulate the unfolded protein response by a direct interaction with IRE1α. Science (New York, N.Y.). 2006;**312**(5773):572-576

[177] Oakes SA, Scorrano L, Opferman JT, Bassik MC, Nishino M, Pozzan T, et al. Proapoptotic BAX and BAK regulate the type 1 inositol trisphosphate receptor and calcium leak from the endoplasmic reticulum. Proceedings of the National Academy of Sciences of the United States of America. 2005;**102**(1):105-110

[178] Deniaud A, Sharaf el dein O, Maillier E, Poncet D, Kroemer G, Lemaire C, et al. Endoplasmic reticulum stress induces calcium-dependent permeability transition, mitochondrial outer membrane permeabilization and apoptosis. Oncogene. 2008;**27**(3):285-299

[179] Luciani DS, Gwiazda KS, T-LB Y, Kalynyak TB, Bychkivska Y, Frey MH, et al. Roles of IP 3 R and RyR Ca 2+ channels in endoplasmic reticulum stress and β-cell death. Diabetes. 2009;**58**(2):422-432

[180] Chami M, Oulès B, Szabadkai G, Tacine R, Rizzuto R, Paterlini-Bréchot P. Role of SERCA1 truncated isoform in the proapoptotic calcium transfer from ER to mitochondria during ER stress. Molecular Cell. 2008;**32**(5):641-651

[181] Csordas G, Renken C, Varnai P, Walter L, Weaver D, Buttle KF, et al. Structural and functional features and significance of the physical linkage between ER and mitochondria. The Journal of Cell Biology. 2006;**174**(7):915-921

[182] Rizzuto R, Pinton P, Carrington W, Fay FS, Fogarty KE, Lifshitz LM, et al. Close contacts with the endoplasmic reticulum as determinants of mitochondrial Ca2+ responses. Science (New York, N.Y.). 1998;**280**(5370):1763-1766

[183] Huang Y, He S, Li JZ, Seo Y-K, Osborne TF, Cohen JC, et al. A feed-forward loop amplifies nutritional regulation of PNPLA3. Proceedings of the National Academy of Sciences. 2010;**107**(17):7892-7897

[184] He S, McPhaul C, Li JZ, Garuti R, Kinch L, Grishin NV, et al. A sequence variation (I148M) in PNPLA3 associated with nonalcoholic fatty liver disease disrupts triglyceride hydrolysis. The Journal of Biological Chemistry. 2010;**285**(9):6706-6715

[185] Valenti L, Alisi A, Galmozzi E, Bartuli A, Del Menico B, Alterio A, et al. I148M patatin-like phospholipase domain-containing 3 gene variant and severity of pediatric nonalcoholic fatty liver disease. Hepatology (Baltimore, Md). 2010;**52**(4):1274-1280

[186] Li YY. Genetic and epigenetic variants influencing the development of nonalcoholic fatty liver disease. World journal of gastroenterology: WJG. 2012;**18**(45):6546

[187] Cheung O, Puri P, Eicken C, Contos MJ, Mirshahi F, Maher JW, et al. Nonalcoholic steatohepatitis is associated with altered hepatic MicroRNA expression. Hepatology. 2008;**48**(6):1810-1820

[188] Esau C, Davis S, Murray SF, XX Y, Pandey SK, Pear M, et al. miR-122 regulation of lipid metabolism revealed by in vivo antisense targeting. Cell Metabolism. 2006;**3**(2):87-98

[189] Krutzfeldt J, Rajewsky N, Braich R, Rajeev KG, Tuschl T, Manoharan M, et al. Silencing of microRNAs in vivo with 'antagomirs. Nature. 2005;**438**(7068):685-689

[190] Sookoian S, Rosselli MS, Gemma C, Burgueno AL, Fernandez Gianotti T, Castano GO, et al. Epigenetic regulation of insulin resistance in nonalcoholic fatty liver disease: Impact of liver methylation of the peroxisome proliferator-activated receptor gamma coactivator 1alpha promoter. Hepatology (Baltimore, Md). 2010;**52**(6):1992-2000

Chapter 3

Role of Lipid Droplet Proteins in the Development of NAFLD and Hepatic Insulin Resistance

Kaori Minehira and Philippe Gual

Additional information is available at the end of the chapter

http://dx.doi.org/10.5772/intechopen.71572

Abstract

NAFLD is diagnosed, when the liver fat exceeds more than 5% of liver weight. Inside of hepatocytes, these fats are stored in cytosolic lipid droplets. The lipid droplets can be formed from a bud, vesicles of the lipid bilayer, which lines at a vicinity of the endoplasmic reticulum (ER). On the surface of droplets, there are several structural/functional proteins such as lipid droplet proteins, lipogenic enzymes, and lipases. Interestingly, the lipid droplet proteins seem to have great impact on a development of NAFLD. Some proteins can interact with transcriptional factors such as SREBP1c and PPAR-alpha/gamma, and some proteins strongly impact a mitochondrial structure. As a result, the lipid droplet proteins highly influence lipid handling and fatty acid oxidation in hepatocytes. This chapter will elucidate our recent understanding of the role of each lipid droplet protein in fatty liver formation and in hepatic insulin resistance. Existing information on genetically modified animals as well as on human NAFLD was reviewed on Perilipin families, CIDE proteins, Seipin, and PNPLAs. Finally, the chapter will discuss how the lipid droplet proteins could potentially lead/protect from hepatic insulin resistance via abnormal accumulation of ceramides and diacylglycerols, autophagy, ER stress, and oxidative stress.

Keywords: perilipin, CIDE proteins, insulin sensitivity, mitochondrial oxidation, autophagy, ER stress

1. Introduction

Liver can store a certain amount of excess glucose as a form of glycogen. A part of the stored glycogen can then be retransformed into glucose (so-called gluconeogenesis) during a fasting condition to leave the liver. Contrary to the glucose, an excess lipid is not normally stored in the liver. However, in a pathological case, excess lipid storage can be observed in hepatocytes, which is called hepatic steatosis. Hepatic steatosis could be diagnosed in different grades according to histological observation (Grade 1: 5–33% lipid invasion in hepatocytes, Grade 2: 33–66%, and Grade 3: >66%). Up to 90% of obese patients could have the hepatic steatosis, and the presence is linked to several metabolic dysfunctions such as insulin resistance, oxidative stress, endoplasmic reticulum (ER) stress, and mitochondrial dysfunctions [1–3]. As a result, hepatic steatosis often leads to abnormal gluconeogenesis, which is a typical phenotype of type 2 diabetes. To better prevent such metabolic dysfunctions, scientists have been actively investigating mechanisms by which hepatic lipids impact metabolic functions.

2. Lipid droplet structure

When excess fat is present in a liver, these fats are stored intracellularly in cytosolic lipid droplet compartment. Today, an origin of a lipid droplet biosynthesis has not been understood completely. Walther and Farese suggested different models of the lipid droplet biosynthesis [4]. Most accepted lipid droplet biosynthesis model is that triglyceride (TG) accumulated at the ER membranes forms a bud, a vesicle of the lipid bilayer [5]. On ER membranes, phospholipids are added onto the surface of growing lipid droplets. Secondary, lipid droplets could increase their size via lipid droplet fusion. Finally, a matured lipid droplet is formed consisting TG and cholesterol esters in a core, coated by a membrane monolayer of phospholipids and sphingomyelin (**Figure 1A**). On the surface and/or vicinity of droplets, there are several structural/functional proteins such as lipid

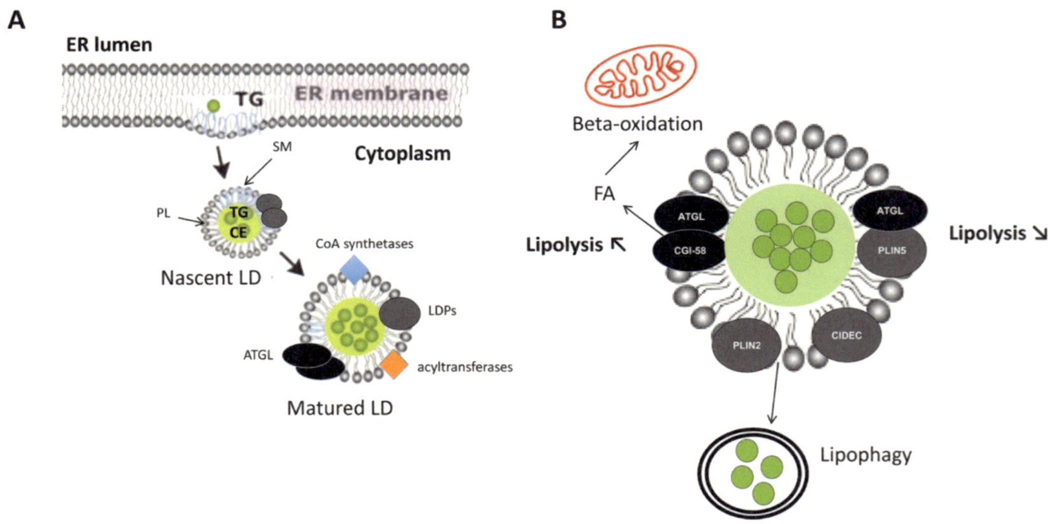

Figure 1. Lipid droplet formation. (A) Formation of nascent lipid droplet (LD) with lipid droplet proteins (LDPs), (B) lipid droplet biology.

http://dx.doi.org/10.5772/intechopen.71572

droplet proteins, lipogenic enzymes, and lipases (**Figure 1B**). Enzymes required for lipid droplet synthesis are also located in the ER. This strategic enzyme location helps to form, stabilize, and degrade lipid droplets when necessary. Hydrolysis of lipid is highly regulated by different enzymes such as adipose triglyceride lipase (ATGL), hormone-sensitive lipase (HSL), and monoglyceride lipase (MGL). ATGL is responsible for the hydrolysis of triglyceride, followed by HSL, which cleaves one molecule of fatty acid from diacylglycerol, and finally hydrolysis is completed by MGL. In hepatocytes, ATGL interacts both lipid droplet protein, perilipin 5 (PLIN5) and comparative gene identification-58 (CGI-58). When ATGL interacts with PLIN5, this decreases lipolysis; however, if ATGL interacts with CGI-58, this increases lipolysis [6]. Therefore, lipid droplet proteins play a key role regulating a fate of cellular lipid storage (**Table 1**).

LD protein	Expression cites	Observed functions	Reported interactions with other genes/proteins
PLIN1 (perilipin A)	WAT, cardiac muscle liposarcoma, BAT	LD stability, control of hormone-induced lipolysis	ATGL, CGI58, [97, 98], SREBP1c [19], CIDEC [15]
PLIN2 (ADRP, adipophilin)	Liver, WAT, mammary gland, macrophages, sebocytes, ubiquitous expression	LD stability, adipocytes differentiation, VLDL lipidation	PPAR alpha, gamma [21, 99, 100], delta [101] hepatic von Hippel-Lindau protein [102]
PLIN3 (TIP47)	Ubiquitous expression, skeletal muscle, neutrophils, sebocytes	LD stability, PGE_2 production, intracellular trafficking	Mannose-6-phosphate receptor [9]
PLIN4 (S3-12)	WAT, skeletal muscle	LD stability, adipocytes differentiation	PLIN5 [32]
PLIN5 (OXPAT, LSDP5, MLDP)	Skeletal muscle, BAT, heart, liver, beta-cells	LD stability, fat oxidation, mitochondrial recruitment	PPARalpha [60], delta [103], CIG58, ATGL [6], ABHD5 [104]
PLPNA3 (Adiponutrin)	WAT, liver, skeletal muscle, pancreas	Triglyceride and retinyl palmitate esterase activity	SREBP1c [105]
PLPNA2 (ATGL)	Adipose tissue	Lipolysis	SIRT1 [106], PLIN5 [6], PLIN1 [33, 97]
CIDEA	Adipose tissue, liver	Lipogenesis	SREBP1c [41, 42]
CIDEB	Adipose tissue	Contributes to lipogenesis, lipidation of VLDL, hepatitis virus assembly	HCV NS58 protein [107]
CIDEC (FSP27)	Adipose tissue, liver	LD stability, LF fusion, lipid transfer	PPAR alpha, gamma [42, 45]
SEIPIN (BCSL)	Adipose tissue, liver, brain, testis	Maturation of LD, lipolysis	

Table 1. Lipid droplet proteins.

3. Lipid droplet protein families

Lipid droplet proteins were discovered in the 1990s in phospholipid monolayer of lipid droplet [7–9]. At that time, each lipid droplet proteins had a different nomenclature. In 2010, it was suggested to uniform their names as the "perilipin family protein: PAT protein" [10]. PAT was named after the three proteins: PLIN1 (Perilipin), PLIN2 (Adipose differentiation-related protein; ADRP), and PLIN3 (Tail-interacting protein of 47 kDa; TIP47). All PLIN families contain a conserved domain called PAT domain [11] with an exception of PLIN4 that only contains long 11-mer repeat motifs [12]. The expression of these proteins and their functions are slightly different, and their exact roles for each cell type have not been yet completely understood. Interestingly, their expression depends on a size of lipid droplets (small lipid droplets: PLIN3, PLIN4, PLIN5; medium lipid droplets: PLIN2; and large lipid droplet: PLIN1).

3.1. PLIN1

PLIN1 was one of the first lipid droplet protein identified in adipocytes [13, 14], and its expression is mainly observed in matured adipocytes. During a differentiation of premature adipocytes, PLIN2 plays a major role to lipidate small lipid droplets. Once lipid droplet gains enough size, PLIN1 replaces PLIN2 to stabilize large lipid-rich lipid droplets and helps to mature adipocytes. PLIN1 also interacts with cell-death-inducing DNA-fragmentation-factor 45-like effector (CIDE)-C for a lipid droplets fusion process [15]. Among different reported functions of PLIN1 in adipocytes, the most well-characterized role of PLIN1 is a control of lipolysis. PLIN1 co-localizes with ATGL and CGI-58 on a surface of lipid droplets at a basal condition. Upon a lipolytic stimulation, PLIN1 is phosphorylated and CGI-58 is released and activates ATGL for a lipolysis. In hepatocytes, PLIN1 is not expressed in normal healthy liver, but its expression is observed in steatotic hepatocytes [16–18]. During a formation of hepatic steatosis, the expression of PLIN1 is synchronized with sterol regulatory element-binding protein (SREBP)-1c, a key regulator of *de novo* lipogenesis [19]. As a result, both genes could strongly contribute to accelerate the pathogenesis of hepatic steatosis [20].

3.2. PLIN2

PLIN2 was originally named as adipose differentiation-related protein due to its high expression during an adipocyte differentiation [8]. PLIN2 is ubiquitously expressed and its expression in the liver is high among other lipid droplet proteins [21]. Chronic alcohol consumption stimulates *de novo* lipogenesis and induces hepatic steatosis together with an upregulation of PLIN2 [22]. Hepatocellular ballooning and oxidative injury were also observed under such condition [18]. Magne et al. observed in human NAFLD patients that PLIN2 polymorphism (ser1Pro) was linked to a decreased VLDL levels [23].

A recent study demonstrated that the PLIN2 and PLIN3 double-knockout in hepatocytes induced insulin resistance [24]. In addition, the overexpression of PLIN2 in rat skeletal muscle resulted in an accumulation of TG in muscle without insulin resistance [25]. However, general deletion of PLIN2 in mice also showed a protective role against hepatic steatosis and insulin resistance (discussed in a later paragraph, **Table 2**). The exact impacts of PLIN2 modification on insulin resistance have not yet been fully elucidated.

LD proteins	Up or downregulation	Outcomes
PLIN1	**Downregulation** KO mice [61] KO mice [62]	Body fat↓, fat oxidation↑ Lipolysis↑, cardiac steatosis↑, cardiac hypertrophy
PLIN2	**Downregulation** ASO [63, 64] KO—alcohol diet [66] KO—high fat diet [65] Liver specific KO—methionine-choline deficient diet [95] Lep (ob/ob)/Plin2 double KO mice [108] KO–high fat diet [109]	Hepatic steatosis↓ (ceramide-, DAG↓), IR ↓ Hepatic steatosis↓ (ceramide↓), IR ↓, glucose tolerance- Hepatic steatosis↓, body fat↓, adipose inflammation↓ Hepatic steatosis↓, hepatic inflammation↓, fibrosis↓ VLDL secretion ↑ Hepatic steatosis ↓, IR↓ (liver, muscle) Hepatic steatosis ↓VLDL -
PLIN3	**Downregulation** ASO [67]	Hepatic steatosis ↓ IR↓
PLIN4	**Downregulation** KO [32]	Cardiac steatosis↓
PLIN5	**Downregulation** KO [38] KO [40] **Upregulation** Adenovirus [68]	Lack of lipid droplet in heart, ROS↑, heart mal function, Hepatic steatosis ↓, mitochondrial oxidative capacity↑, lipotoxic injury Hepatic steatosis ↑ IR-
PLPNA3	**Downregulation** KO [55, 56] **Upregulation** G allele knock-in Ref. [57]	Hepatic steatosis - Hepatic steatosis ↑
PLPNA2	**Downregulation** KO [69] Liver-specific KO [70]	Steatosis in different organs↑, IR↓ Hepatic steatosis ↑ (DAG↓), IR -
CIDEC	**Downregulation** KO [47, 110] KO in ob/ob by shRNA [46] ASO [111] **Upregulation** Adenovirus [46]	Hepatic steatosis ↓, IR↓ Hepatic steatosis ↓, IR↓ Hepatic steatosis ↓, body fat↓, IR↓ Hepatic steatosis↑
SEIPIN	**Downregulation** Adipose-specific KO [112] KO [49] **Upregulation** Transgenic mice overexpressing a short isoform of human BSCL2 in adipose [113]	Hepatic steatosis↑, IR↑, adipocyte hypertrophy and progressive lipodystrophy Hepatic steatosis↑, IR↑ Hepatic steatosis↑, IR↑, white adipose tissue ↓, lipolysis ↑

Abbreviations: KO; knockout, ASO; antisense oligonucleotide, IR; insulin resistance.

Table 2. Experimental modification of lipid droplet protein and the effect on steatosis.

3.3. PLIN3

PLIN3 was originally named tail-interacting protein of 47 kDa and ubiquitously expressed among tissues. PLIN3 is localized at the cytosol and lipid droplet [9, 26]. It is also implicated in intracellular trafficking of lysosomal enzymes [9]. Four-helix bundle in PLIN3 has been suggested to contribute to fatty acid binding and lipid droplet recruitment [9]. PLIN2 and PLIN3 share similar functions, and both proteins cannot bind CGI-58 and, therefore, influence lipolysis [27]. Co-expression of PLIN2 and PLIN3 has been reported in many tissues; however, a distinct role of PLIN3 has not been clearly identified. Interestingly, PLIN3 expression was also observed in stellate cells in the liver [17]. Lipopolysaccharide treatment also predominantly stimulated PLIN3 expression in HL-60-derived neutrophils [28]. Knockdown of PLIN3 via siRNA decreased a lipid droplet formation as well as PGE_2 secretion. This observation was unique to PLIN3, and PLIN2 was not detected under such conditions. This implies that PLIN3 might be implicated in a lipid droplet formation related to conditions with cellular stresses.

Another unique observation to PLIN3 was that mice lacking mTORC2 (mammalian target of rapamycin complex) activity in skeletal muscle showed increased fat mass and PLIN3 [29]. This was due to an increased AMPK activity. mTORC plays an important role in insulin signaling. However, the implication of PLIN3 in insulin resistance has not yet been addressed.

3.4. PLIN4

PLIN4 was originally called S3–12 and is the only PAT protein that does not contain the PAT domain. Its molecular weight is three times higher than other PAT proteins. The protein has been shown to present at cytosol and lipid droplets [30]. Its expression was induced during adipogenesis [31]. PLIN4-KO mice present no phenotypic changes in adipose tissues, whereas TG content in heart tissues was significantly reduced [32]. PLIN5 expression was also decreased under such condition. Given close location of PLIN4 and PLIN5 in chromosome 19 in human, it was suggested a potential transcriptional interference between two genes. PLIN4 remains the least studied PAT protein, and further investigations are required to understand PLIN4 roles in lipid droplet physiology.

3.5. PLIN5

PLIN5 was discovered by different researchers simultaneously and named as myocardial lipid droplet protein (MDLP), OXPAT, or lipid storage droplet protein 5 (LSDP5) [33, 34]. This was due to a high expression of PLIN5 in heart and other oxidative tissues such as skeletal muscle and liver. PLIN5 expression is also reported in pancreatic beta cells and hepatic stellate cells [35, 36]. A unique feature with PLIN5 is that mitochondria are physically recruited to lipid droplets expressing high PLIN5 (**Figure 2**) [37, 38]. Its expression is regulated by PPAR-alpha, and most importantly, PLIN5 plays roles in regulating cellular fat oxidation. PLIN5 stabilizes lipid droplets by sequestrating fatty acids, and because PLIN5 can recruit mitochondria to lipid droplet surface, it facilitates to release fatty acids to mitochondria for the oxidation [39]. Given its gatekeeper roles on the lipid oxidation, it has been suggested that PLIN5 could protect cardiac myocytes and hepatocytes from oxidative stress [38, 40]. PLIN5 leads several modifications on the lipid metabolism as well as insulin sensitivity, and details are discussed in a separate paragraph.

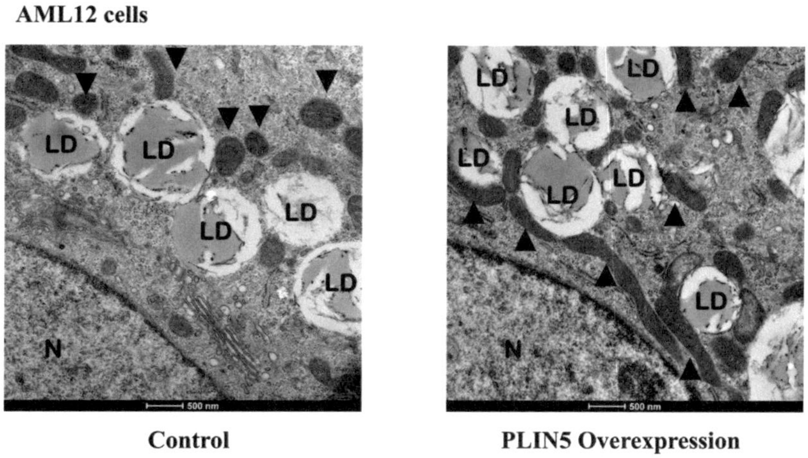

Figure 2. Electron microscopy image of hepatocyte overexpressing PLIN5. When PLIN5 is overexpressed, mitochondria (closed triangle) is highly recruited toward lipid droplets (LD). N: nucleus.

3.6. CIDE proteins

Cell-death-inducing DNA fragmentation-factor 45-like effector (CIDE) proteins have also been found on a lipid droplet surface. CIDEA expression is controlled by SREBP-1c and found in a fatty liver [41, 42]. CIDEB is constitutively expressed in a liver and plays a role in VLDL production [43, 44]. Interestingly, it has been reported that CIDEB and PLIN2 exert opposite functions for a control of VLDL lipidation [44]. CIDEC, is also named as fat-specific protein 27 (FSP27), found as a cofactor of PLIN1 for lipid droplet fusion in adipocytes [15]. CIDEC is regulated by PPAR-alpha/gamma [42, 45]. Like CIDEA, hepatic CIDEC was induced in leptin-deficient *ob/ob* mice. It has also been demonstrated that CIDEC overexpression induces steatosis, whereas knockdown of CIDEC alleviates hepatic fat accumulation in *ob/ob* mice lacking hepatic PPARγ [46]. Effect of CIDEC on mitochondrial activity and insulin sensitivity is an active research field of today [15, 47, 48]. Toy et al. demonstrated that white adipocytes from CIDEC KO mice had accelerated mitochondrial activities and increased proteins and size, leading to brown adipocyte characteristics.

3.7. SEIPIN

SEIPIN is highly expressed in brain, testis, and adipose tissue. Mutations in SEIPIN are known as Berardinelli-Seip congenital lipodystrophy (BSCL), a rare recessive disorder characterized by near absence of adipose tissue accompanied by a severe insulin resistance [49]. Several studies convincingly demonstrated that SEIPIN plays a crucial role in adipogenesis, lipid droplet homeostasis and lipolysis. It is also well known that human BSCL patients and mice lacking SEIPIN develop diabetes and severe hepatic steatosis. Interestingly, our previous studies demonstrated that SEIPIN expression seems to be dependent on lipid droplet size (**Figure 3**), and the low SEIPIN expresser had an impaired gluconeogenesis in NAFLD patients (personal observation).

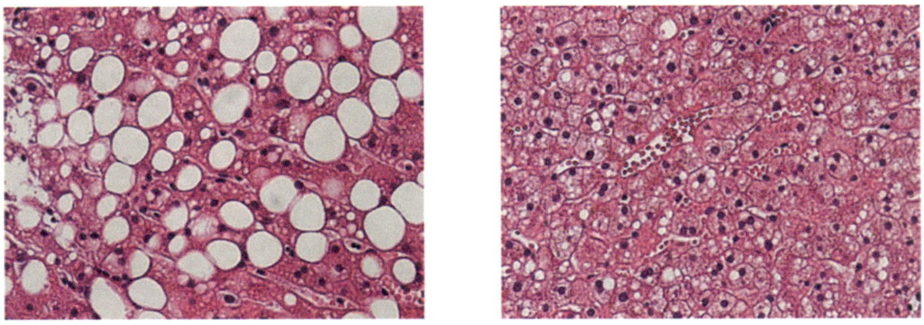

Figure 3. Liver histology from NAFLD patients.

3.8. PNPLA3 and PNPLA2

Patatin-like phospholipase domain-containing protein 3 (PNPLA3), also called adiponutrin, was consistently associated with NAFLD in GWAS observations [50, 51]. The single nucleotide polymorphism (SNP) in PNPLA3 was identified as a major determinant of hepatic fat content from exome-wide association studies. This is the rs738409 C > G SNP encoding for the isoleucine to methionine substitution [50]. PNPLA3 is expressed in the retina, hepatic stellate cells, and hepatocytes and localized in the endoplasmic reticulum and at a surface of lipid droplets. A mechanism by which PNPLA3 leads the hepatic steatosis phenotype has not been clearly understood. PNPLA3 has a triglyceride and retinylpalmitate esterase activity [52–54], suggesting a possible link to hepatic fat accumulation. However, PNPLA3 knockout mice did not develop hepatic steatosis [55, 56]. Mice having Pnpla3i148m knock-in recently showed increased hepatic steatosis [57]. The role of PNPLA3 in the development of NAFLD still remains elusive.

PNPLA2 is known as adipose triglyceride transfer protein (ATGL) and is expressed on lipid droplet surface at a basal condition. Its activity is strongly influenced by PLINs [25]. As shown in **Figure 1**, ATGL is the first enzyme hydrolyzing neutral lipids.

4. Expression of lipid droplet proteins in human NAFLD

Lipid droplet proteins are highly expressed in human NAFLD. PLIN1, PLIN2, and PLIN3 were upregulated in NAFLD [18, 58, 59]. And the distribution of PLINs seems to depend on the lipid droplet size [17, 18]. PLIN2 was also observed in stellate cells [18, 59]. We have compared the expression of different lipid droplet proteins in human NAFLD. The steatosis was judged by a histological assessment showing four different grades (S0 < S1 < S2 < S3). Despite a similar BMI among different groups, the gene expression of lipid droplet proteins increased depending on the degree of steatosis (**Figure 4A**). When compared the livers from patients with or without type 2 diabetes who had a similar degree of hepatic steatosis (S3), the expressions of lipid droplet proteins were significantly lower in diabetic patients than in nondiabetic individuals (**Figure 4B**). This result implies possible link between lipid droplet proteins and hepatic insulin signaling.

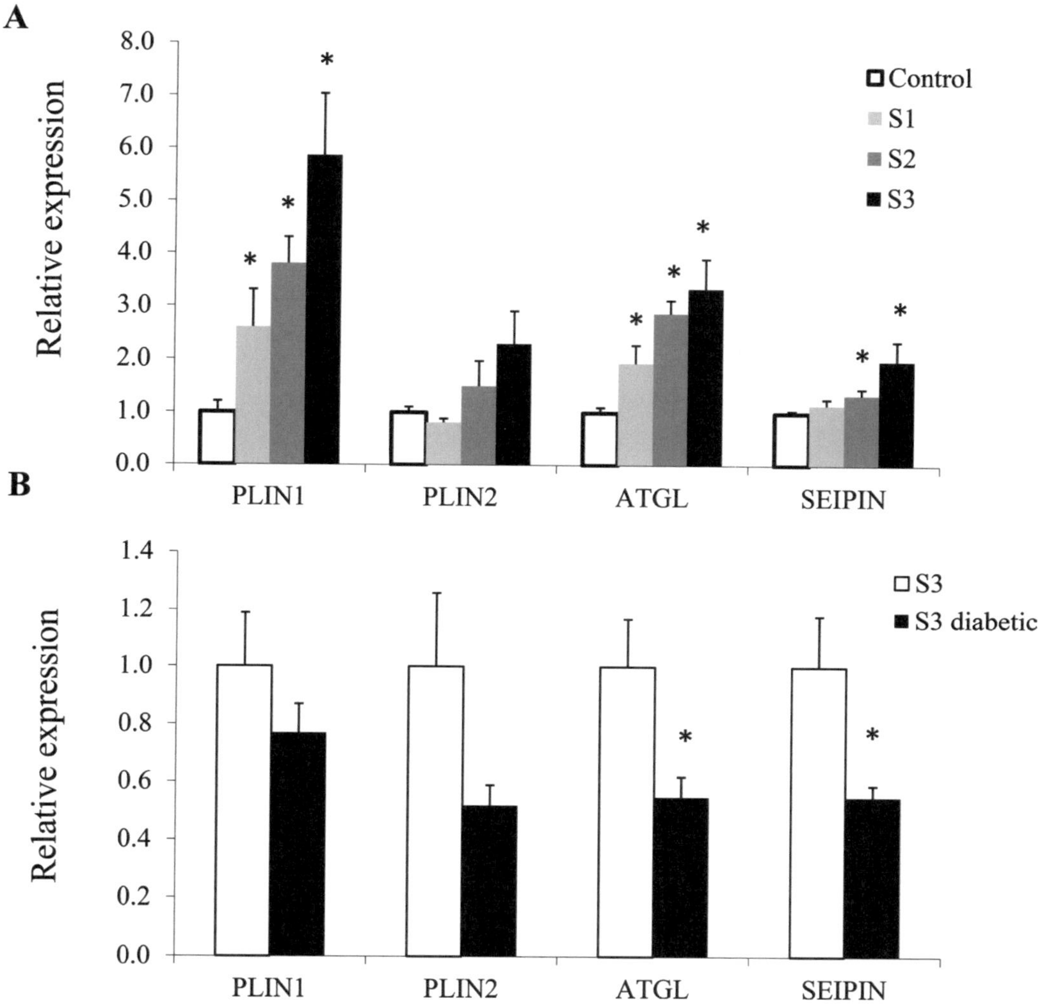

Figure 4. Expression of lipid droplet proteins in human NAFLD. NAFLD patients were separated into 5 groups depending on their degree of fatty liver. Gene expression of lipid droplets genes were analysed and compared among groups. (A) NALFD non diabetic, (B) Comparison of S3 NAFLD patients with or without type 2 diabetes.

5. Experimental modification of lipid droplet proteins and TG accumulation in hepatocytes

It has been shown that modifications on the lipid droplet proteins have striking impacts on lipid droplet biology. Hepatic cell line AML-12 is used to study the effect of downregulation of SEIPIN gene. Downregulation of the gene markedly altered lipid droplets size distributions and increased smaller droplets size, suggesting a default in lipid droplet maturation (**Figure 5**). When PLIN5 was knocked down in hepatocytes, the TG content dramatically

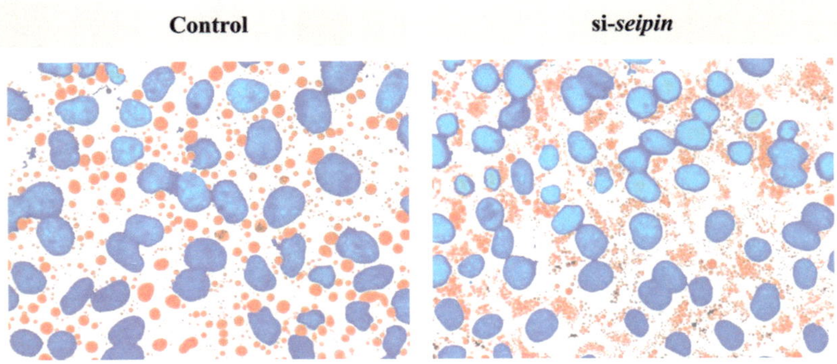

Figure 5. Lipid droplet morphology when SEIPIN was downregulated. Downregulation of SEIPIN by siRNA resulted in a fractionation of lipid droplets.

decreased due to accelerated lipolysis and beta-oxidation [60]. PPAR-alpha was required for the PLIN5-induced beta-oxidation. On the contrary, the overexpression of PLIN5 leads a significant increase in cellular TG. Therefore, modifications on lipid droplets proteins govern intracellular TG content in hepatocytes, although the mechanisms and phenotypes (lipid droplet size and/or localization) might be depending on a type of lipid droplet proteins involved.

6. Experimental modification of lipid droplet proteins in mice

Table 2 displays animals with genetic modifications in lipid droplet proteins and their effect on steatosis and metabolism (**Table 2**). PLIN1 KO mice present reduced body fat as well as fat oxidation judged by respiratory quotient [61]. Another research group also studied the PLIN1 KO mice and found increased lipolysis and cardiac hypertrophy [62]. PLIN2 null mice studied by different scientific groups consistently demonstrated a protection against diet-induced obesity, fatty liver, and alcohol-induced fatty accompanied by an improved insulin sensitivity [63–66]. Similar results were obtained in mice treated by PLIN2 antisense oligonucleotide, demonstrating improved insulin sensitivity [64]. PLIN3 downregulation was studied by using antisense oligonucleotide (ASO) in C57BL/6 J mice fed high fat diet. The reduction in PLIN3 significantly decreased hepatic fat content and improved glucose tolerance as well as insulin sensitivity in liver, adipose, and skeletal muscle [67]. Chen et al. generated PLIN4 KO mice [32], which showed no major modification in body weight and fat mass. Interestingly, only cardiac TG content was significantly reduced. The KO mice did not alter any gene expression involved in glucose and lipid metabolism. PLIN5 KO mice also developed cardiac dysfunction. The PLIN5 KO animal displayed reduced hepatic steatosis with increased mitochondrial proliferation, lipotoxic injury in the hepatocytes [40]. Interestingly, overexpression of PLIN5 by use of adenovirus technology demonstrated a development of severe hepatic steatosis without a sign of hepatic insulin resistance [68].

Although a strong link between PNPLA3 and hepatic steatosis has been demonstrated in GWAS studies [50], absence of PNPLA3 gene did not influence TG hydrolysis, nor did hepatic steatosis [55, 56]. One of a pioneer study on the lipid droplet biology and insulin resistance was the PNPLA2/ATGL KO mice published in 2006 [69]. Mice with global ATGL deletion induced TG accumulation in all tissues [69]. Surprisingly, despite the severe steatosis, the mice exhibit enhanced glucose tolerance and insulin sensitivity. Later on, Wu et al. studied the effect of liver-specific deletion of ATGL [70]. The liver-specific KO mice progressively developed a severe form of hepatic steatosis; however, the hepatic DAG content was 50-fold lower and had comparable plasma glucose, TG, and cholesterol levels to those of controls.

CIDEC/FSP27 downregulation was studied in Fsp27−/− and ob/ob × Fsp27−/− mice [46, 47], demonstrating decreased hepatic steatosis and insulin resistance. These animals are resistant to diet-induced obesity, dyslipidemia. Deletion of SEIPIN, as seen in BSCL patients, leads to severe form of hepatic steatosis accompanied by insulin resistance [49].

7. NAFLD and insulin resistance, implication of lipid droplet proteins

It has been widely accepted that increased TG content in ectopic organs, especially in the liver and skeletal muscle, induces insulin resistance [71–73]. Despite strong evidences demonstrating the link, there are also a few studies to show that hepatic steatosis can be dissociated from

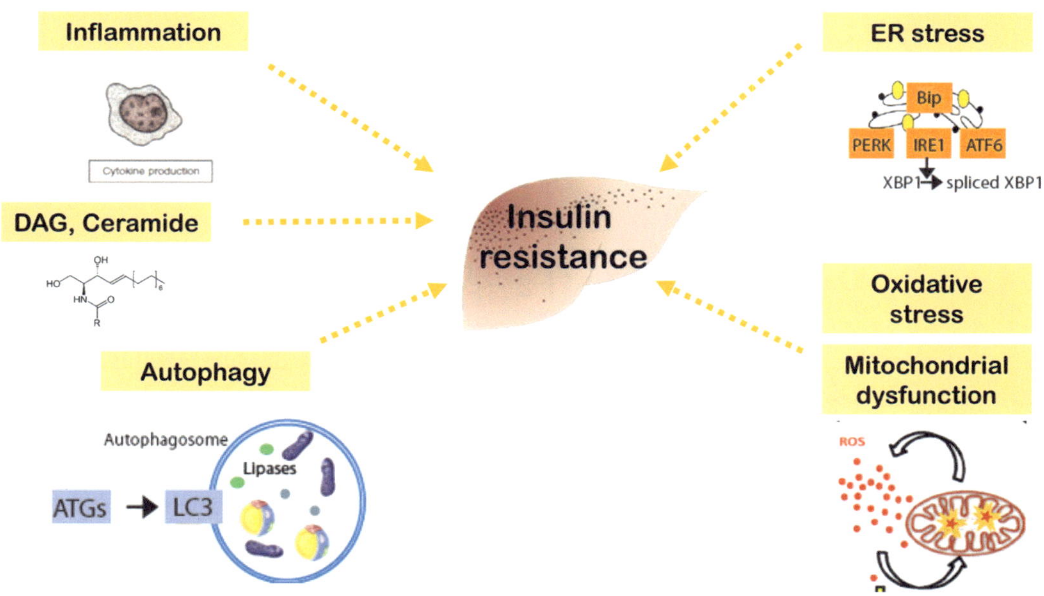

Figure 6. Different events leading hepatic insulin resistance in NAFLD. In human NAFLD, increased diacylglycerols (DAG) and ceramides are often observed. Under such conditions, autophagy is frequently decreased, leading to a disturbed lipid handling as well as increased ER stress and oxidative stress. These factors are known to induce insulin resistance.

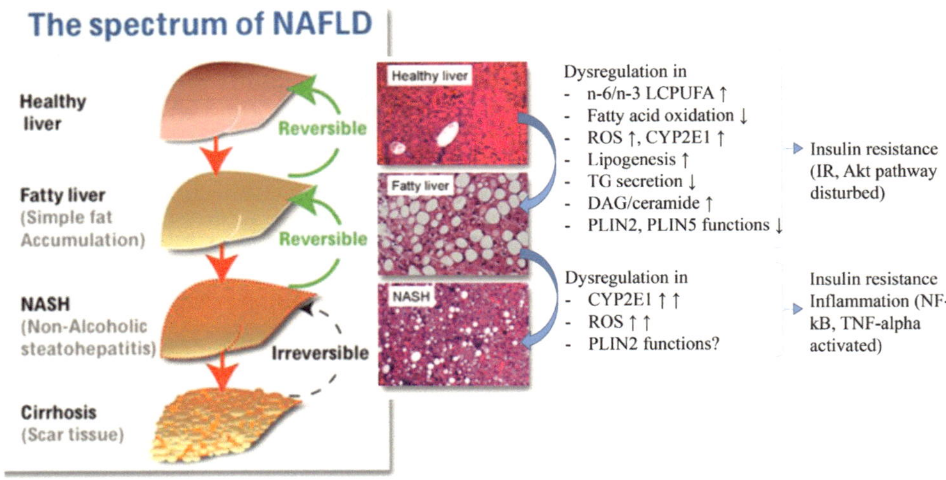

Figure 7. Dysregulated factors during steatosis and NASH development. Hepatic steatosis has many dysregulation in lipid metabolism, leading to insulin resistance. As a result of accelerated cellular damages due to oxidative stress and ER stress, inflammation is installed and NASH development starts.

insulin resistance such as liver-specific microsomal TG transfer protein (MTP) knockout mice [74]. While it is not physiological context at all, it may help to understand the contribution of each gene to the development of hepatic steatosis and insulin resistance at a molecular level. In a steatotic liver from the MTP knockout mice, we had identified upregulations of different lipid droplet proteins such as PLIN5, PLIN2, and SEIPIN. We then hypothesized that the upregulation of these genes was not deleterious in terms of hepatic insulin sensitivity. Indeed, the overexpression of these lipid droplet proteins always induced TG accumulation in hepatocytes; however, none of these *in vitro* models developed apparent insulin resistance. If true, what mechanisms possibly explain the development of hepatic insulin resistance in NAFLD? Different theories are briefly introduced below (**Figures 6** and **7**).

8. Ceramide/Diacylglycerol theory

In a steatotic liver, different lipid species are accumulated such as diacylglycerol (DAG) and ceramide. It was postulated that the accumulation of DAG and/or ceramide induced insulin resistance [75]. However, some of the models of NAFLD present increased hepatic DAG and ceramide without insulin resistance. Interestingly, a recent study demonstrated that the abnormal compartmentalization of these lipid intermediates, rather than total lipid content, is what might truly interfere with the insulin sensitivity [76]. This might support some inconsistent results from various mouse models studied by modulating PLINs (**Table 2**). DAG induces PKC epsilon translocation to the plasma membrane, inhibiting the intracellular kinase domain of the insulin receptor [77, 78]. In the case of PLIN5 overexpressed liver that was dissociated from hepatic insulin resistance, we did not observe the PKC epsilon translocation to the plasma membrane despite significant increase in DAG (personal observation). Accumulation of ceramides in the plasma membrane has also been demonstrated to disturb insulin signaling [79], and we have only observed significant increase in some of ceramides. As the PLIN-induced hepatic steatosis might depend on the type of PLIN proteins, each phenotype of hepatic steatosis needs to be finely studied. Therefore, the link between DAG/ceramide and hepatic insulin resistance in NAFLD requires more scientific investigations on each specific PLIN protein modification.

9. Autophagy theory

Selective autophagy process for a degradation of intracellular lipids is called lipophagy. The lipophagy is an additional mechanism that contributes to lipid droplet breakdown, and PLIN2 has been shown to play a role in this process [80, 81]. Autophagy is also involved in delivering fatty acids to lipid droplets for a lipolysis and mitochondrial oxidation [82, 83]. Inhibition of autophagy has been shown to accelerate lipid accumulation and impair beta-oxidation in the liver [84, 85]. Interestingly, *atg7* inhibition via shRNA in a mouse liver resulted in an impairment of autophagy system together with an impaired insulin signaling and an induced ER stress [85]. These effects were completely reversed when a downstream target *atg5* was blocked. This strongly supports an idea that autophagy plays one of a key role in insulin signaling pathway. How the lipophagy and lipid droplet proteins are involved in the insulin resistance are still open questions.

10. ER stress theory

Hepatic ER deals with redox regulation, glucose deprivation, protein synthesis, VLDL assembly and secretion, and cholesterol biosynthesis. It has been suggested that ER stress is implicated in insulin resistance, inflammation, and lipotoxicity, which are frequently observed in NAFLD patients [86]. Recently, Akoumi et al. tested a hypothesis that palmitate might induce ER stress by disturbing lipid droplet formation in cytosol and lead to an abnormal accumulation of lipid in an ER compartment. They found in cardiomyoblast cell line that palmitate-induced ER stress was associated with an abnormal storage of DAGs located in the ER. Concomitantly, significant degradation of PLIN2 but not PLIN3 or PLIN5 was observed, suggesting a potential scenario of PLIN2 as a protector/regulator of ER stress. Pharmacological ER stress also demonstrated a role of PLIN2 in ER stress-induced lipogenesis [87]. Author suggested that the presence (or induction) of PLIN2 during the ER stress might protect hepatocytes by storing lipids in a cytosolic compartment. It was a very tentative hypothesis; however, it was not supported at least in *Saccharomyces cerevisiae* that an absence of lipid droplet formation did not affect cell viability during ER stress [88]. There are still many remaining questions to be answered in the field of ER stress and the role of lipid droplet proteins. Their implication on metabolic disease such as NAFLD is one of a key aspect to be further investigated.

11. Oxidative stress theory

Reactive oxygen species (ROS) is produced in a highly regulated manner in multiple organelles such as the ER and mitochondria. ROS is produced as a result of oxidative protein folding and mitochondrial respiration. NAFLD, especially NASH (nonalcoholic steatohepatitis), has been strongly linked with the biomarkers of oxidative stress [89, 90]. In a case of NAFLD development, beta-oxidation can be abnormally stimulated due to an excess fat accumulation, which surcharges mitochondrial system for the oxidation. As a result, abnormal ROS production at complex I of the mitochondrial electron-transport chain is induced, leading to the mitochondrial oxidative damage. Under such condition, the redox imbalance, lower antioxidant potential, and an enhanced free-radical activity lead to a significant reduction in systemic antioxidant capacity of plasma [91]. These conditions are indeed considered as a trigger of "second hit," which then induces NASH. Cytochrome P450 E12 (CYP2E1), a member of the cytochrome P450 mixed-function oxidase system, has been found as a marker of NASH, which distinguishes NASH from hepatic steatosis [92]. The induction of liver microsomal CYP2E1 contributes as a major free-radical source that aggravates oxidative stress in NASH. In addition to ROS production, cytokine is produced progressing a fatty liver to NASH. A depletion of *n*-3 long-chain polyunsaturated fatty acids (LCPUFA) was also found in NAFLD/NASH. *n*-3 LCPUFA has been shown to highly influence signaling pathway in a liver and contributes to NAFLD development [93, 94]. The *n*-3 LCPUFA downregulates sterol regulatory element-binding protein-1 (SRBBP-1), therefore inhibiting *de novo* lipogenesis. It could also act as a ligand activators of PPAR-alpha, therefore stimulating fatty acid oxidation. The decreased n-3 LCPUFA and increased ratio of n-6/n-3 LCPUFA were reported in NAFLD/NASH patients. These conditions accelerate high oxidative stress and hepatocellular injury. Interestingly, Fujii et al. demonstrated in NAFLD/NASH patients that PLIN2 seemed preferentially expressed in droplets of ballooned hepatocytes. The presence of PLIN2-positive ballooned hepatocytes was indeed correlated with inflammation [18]. Indeed, liver-specific knockout of PLIN2 in mice had reduced hepatic inflammation [95]. The role of PLIN2 on hepatic inflammation in NAFLD/NASH needs further investigation.

As indicated previously, PLIN5 has strong interactions with mitochondrial functions. Zheng et al. studied myocardium from PLIN5-deficient mice and found that the ROS production and malondialdehyde levels, a marker for oxidative stress, were significantly increased [96]. In this model, the phosphorylation of PI3K and Akt, which was induced by ischemia/reperfusion injury, was greatly reduced by PLIN5 deletion in the myocardium. It remains an open question whether the PLIN5 may have an impact on NASH development by interfering with the ROS production.

12. Conclusion

Research on lipid droplet proteins and lipid droplet biology has gained strong insights during the last decades. Most of the lipid droplet proteins are induced in NAFLD and required for a normal adipogenesis. Given specific expression patterns and roles of lipid droplet proteins, the phenotypes lead by experimental modifications of the lipid droplets proteins displayed diverse patterns. Further research is required to clarify their roles in NAFLD, specially by focusing on interactions of different lipid droplet proteins and other functional

http://dx.doi.org/10.5772/intechopen.71572

proteins, lipid droplet localization, interaction with mitochondria as well as fatty acid compositions in the droplets. Their roles in mitochondrial physiology are a particular importance to understand how lipid droplet protein could influence hepatic energy metabolism and insulin signaling.

Author details

Kaori Minehira[1]* and Philippe Gual[2]

*Address all correspondence to: kaori.minehiracastelli@rd.nestle.com

1 Nestlé Institute of Health Sciences, Lausanne, Switzerland

2 Université Côte d'Azur, INSERM, U1065, C3M, Team 8, Chronic liver diseases associated with obesity and alcohol, Nice, France

References

[1] de Alwis NM, Day CP. Non-alcoholic fatty liver disease: The mist gradually clears. Journal of Hepatology. 2008;**48**(Suppl 1):S104-S112

[2] Kaser S, Ebenbichler CF, Tilg H. Pharmacological and non-pharmacological treatment of non-alcoholic fatty liver disease. International Journal of Clinical Practice. 2010; **64**(7):968-983

[3] Byrne CD, Targher GNAFLD. A multisystem disease. Journal of Hepatology. 2015; **62**(1 Suppl):S47-S64

[4] Farese RV Jr, Walther TC. Lipid droplets finally get a little R-E-S-P-E-C-T. Cell. 2009; **139**(5):855-860

[5] Tan JS, Seow CJ, Goh VJ, Silver DL. Recent advances in understanding proteins involved in lipid droplet formation, growth and fusion. Journal of Genetics and Genomics. 2014;**41**(5):251-259

[6] Wang H, Bell M, Sreenivasan U, Hu H, Liu J, Dalen K, et al. Unique regulation of adipose triglyceride lipase (ATGL) by perilipin 5, a lipid droplet-associated protein. The Journal of Biological Chemistry. 2011;**286**(18):15707-15715

[7] Greenberg AS, Egan JJ, Wek SA, Garty NB, Blanchette-Mackie EJ, Londos C. Perilipin, a major hormonally regulated adipocyte-specific phosphoprotein associated with the periphery of lipid storage droplets. The Journal of Biological Chemistry. 1991;**266**(17): 11341-11346

[8] Jiang HP, Serrero G. Isolation and characterization of a full-length cDNA coding for an adipose differentiation-related protein. Proceedings of the National Academy of Sciences of the United States of America. 1992;**89**(17):7856-7860

[9] Diaz E, Pfeffer SR. TIP47: A cargo selection device for mannose 6-phosphate receptor trafficking. Cell. 1998;**93**(3):433-443

[10] Kimmel AR, Brasaemle DL, McAndrews-Hill M, Sztalryd C, Londos C. Adoption of PERILIPIN as a unifying nomenclature for the mammalian PAT-family of intracellular lipid storage droplet proteins. Journal of Lipid Research. 2010;**51**(3):468-471

[11] Miura S, Gan JW, Brzostowski J, Parisi MJ, Schultz CJ, Londos C, et al. Functional conservation for lipid storage droplet association among Perilipin, ADRP, and TIP47 (PAT)-related proteins in mammals, drosophila, and Dictyostelium. The Journal of Biological Chemistry. 2002;**277**(35):32253-32257

[12] Itabe H, Yamaguchi T, Nimura S, Sasabe N. Perilipins: A diversity of intracellular lipid droplet proteins. Lipids in Health and Disease. 2017;**16**(1):83

[13] Brasaemle DL, Rubin B, Harten IA, Gruia-Gray J, Kimmel AR, Londos C. Perilipin a increases triacylglycerol storage by decreasing the rate of triacylglycerol hydrolysis. The Journal of Biological Chemistry. 2000;**275**(49):38486-38493

[14] Blanchette-Mackie EJ, Dwyer NK, Barber T, Coxey RA, Takeda T, Rondinone CM, et al. Perilipin is located on the surface layer of intracellular lipid droplets in adipocytes. Journal of Lipid Research. 1995;**36**(6):1211-1226

[15] Sun Z, Gong J, Wu H, Xu W, Wu L, Xu D, et al. Perilipin1 promotes unilocular lipid droplet formation through the activation of Fsp27 in adipocytes. Nature Communications. 2013;**4**:1594

[16] Caldwell SH, Ikura Y, Iezzoni JC, Liu Z. Has natural selection in human populations produced two types of metabolic syndrome (with and without fatty liver)? Journal of Gastroenterology and Hepatology. 2007;**22**(Suppl 1):S11-S19

[17] Straub BK, Stoeffel P, Heid H, Zimbelmann R, Schirmacher P. Differential pattern of lipid droplet-associated proteins and de novo perilipin expression in hepatocyte steatogenesis. Hepatology. 2008;**47**(6):1936-1946

[18] Fujii H, Ikura Y, Arimoto J, Sugioka K, Iezzoni JC, Park SH, et al. Expression of perilipin and adipophilin in nonalcoholic fatty liver disease; relevance to oxidative injury and hepatocyte ballooning. Journal of Atherosclerosis and Thrombosis. 2009;**16**(6):893-901

[19] Takahashi Y, Shinoda A, Furuya N, Harada E, Arimura N, Ichi I, et al. Perilipin-mediated lipid droplet formation in adipocytes promotes sterol regulatory element-binding protein-1 processing and triacylglyceride accumulation. PLoS One. 2013;**8**(5):e64605

[20] Beier JI, McClain CJ. Mechanisms and cell signaling in alcoholic liver disease. Biological Chemistry. 2010;**391**(11):1249-1264

[21] Motomura W, Inoue M, Ohtake T, Takahashi N, Nagamine M, Tanno S, et al. Up-regulation of ADRP in fatty liver in human and liver steatosis in mice fed with high fat diet. Biochemical and Biophysical Research Communications. 2006;**340**(4):1111-1118

[22] Carr RM, Dhir R, Yin X, Agarwal B, Ahima RS. Temporal effects of ethanol consumption on energy homeostasis, hepatic steatosis, and insulin sensitivity in mice. Alcoholism, Clinical and Experimental Research. 2013;**37**(7):1091-1099

[23] Magne J, Aminoff A, Perman Sundelin J, Mannila MN, Gustafsson P, Hultenby K, et al. The minor allele of the missense polymorphism Ser251Pro in perilipin 2 (PLIN2) disrupts an alpha-helix, affects lipolysis, and is associated with reduced plasma triglyceride concentration in humans. The FASEB Journal. 2013;**27**(8):3090-3099

[24] Bell M, Wang H, Chen H, McLenithan JC, Gong DW, Yang RZ, et al. Consequences of lipid droplet coat protein downregulation in liver cells: Abnormal lipid droplet metabolism and induction of insulin resistance. Diabetes. 2008;**57**(8):2037-2045

[25] Coleman RA, Mashek DG. Mammalian triacylglycerol metabolism: Synthesis, lipolysis, and signaling. Chemical Reviews. 2011;**111**(10):6359-6386

[26] Lu X, Gruia-Gray J, Copeland NG, Gilbert DJ, Jenkins NA, Londos C, et al. The murine perilipin gene: The lipid droplet-associated perilipins derive from tissue-specific, mRNA splice variants and define a gene family of ancient origin. Mammalian Genome. 2001;**12**(9):741-749

[27] Patel S, Yang W, Kozusko K, Saudek V, Savage DB. Perilipins 2 and 3 lack a carboxy-terminal domain present in perilipin 1 involved in sequestering ABHD5 and suppressing basal lipolysis. Proceedings of the National Academy of Sciences of the United States of America. 2014;**111**(25):9163-9168

[28] Nose F, Yamaguchi T, Kato R, Aiuchi T, Obama T, Hara S, et al. Crucial role of perilipin-3 (TIP47) in formation of lipid droplets and PGE2 production in HL-60-derived neutrophils. PLoS One. 2013;**8**(8):e71542

[29] Kleinert M, Parker BL, Chaudhuri R, Fazakerley DJ, Serup A, Thomas KC, et al. mTORC2 and AMPK differentially regulate muscle triglyceride content via Perilipin 3. Molecular Metabolism. 2016;**5**(8):646-655

[30] Wolins NE, Skinner JR, Schoenfish MJ, Tzekov A, Bensch KG, Bickel PE. Adipocyte protein S3-12 coats nascent lipid droplets. The Journal of Biological Chemistry. 2003;**278**(39):37713-37721

[31] Nimura S, Yamaguchi T, Ueda K, Kadokura K, Aiuchi T, Kato R, et al. Olanzapine promotes the accumulation of lipid droplets and the expression of multiple perilipins in human adipocytes. Biochemical and Biophysical Research Communications. 2015;**467**(4):906-912

[32] Chen W, Chang B, Wu X, Li L, Sleeman M, Chan L. Inactivation of Plin4 downregulates Plin5 and reduces cardiac lipid accumulation in mice. American Journal of Physiology. Endocrinology and Metabolism. 2013;**304**(7):E770-E779

[33] Yamaguchi T, Matsushita S, Motojima K, Hirose F, Osumi TMLDP. A novel PAT family protein localized to lipid droplets and enriched in the heart, is regulated by peroxisome proliferator-activated receptor alpha. The Journal of Biological Chemistry. 2006;**281**(20):14232-14240

[34] Dalen KT, Dahl T, Holter E, Arntsen B, Londos C, Sztalryd C, et al. LSDP5 is a PAT protein specifically expressed in fatty acid oxidizing tissues. Biochimica et Biophysica Acta. 2007;**1771**(2):210-227

[35] Trevino MB, Machida Y, Hallinger DR, Garcia E, Christensen A, Dutta S, et al. Perilipin 5 regulates islet lipid metabolism and insulin secretion in a cAMP-dependent manner: Implication of its role in the postprandial insulin secretion. Diabetes. 2015;**64**(4): 1299-1310

[36] Lin J, Chen A. Perilipin 5 restores the formation of lipid droplets in activated hepatic stellate cells and inhibits their activation. Laboratory Investigation. 2016;**96**(7):791-806

[37] Bosma M, Minnaard R, Sparks LM, Schaart G, Losen M, de Baets MH, et al. The lipid droplet coat protein perilipin 5 also localizes to muscle mitochondria. Histochemistry and Cell Biology. 2012;**137**(2):205-216

[38] Kuramoto K, Okamura T, Yamaguchi T, Nakamura TY, Wakabayashi S, Morinaga H, et al. Perilipin 5, a lipid droplet-binding protein, protects heart from oxidative burden by sequestering fatty acid from excessive oxidation. The Journal of Biological Chemistry. 2012;**287**(28):23852-23863

[39] Wang H, Sreenivasan U, Hu H, Saladino A, Polster BM, Lund LM, et al. Perilipin 5, a lipid droplet-associated protein, provides physical and metabolic linkage to mitochondria. Journal of Lipid Research. 2011;**52**(12):2159-2168

[40] Wang C, Zhao Y, Gao X, Li L, Yuan Y, Liu F, et al. Perilipin 5 improves hepatic lipotoxicity by inhibiting lipolysis. Hepatology. 2015;**61**(3):870-882

[41] Wang R, Kong X, Cui A, Liu X, Xiang R, Yang Y, et al. Sterol-regulatory-element-binding protein 1c mediates the effect of insulin on the expression of Cidea in mouse hepatocytes. The Biochemical Journal. 2010;**430**(2):245-254

[42] Zhou L, Xu L, Ye J, Li D, Wang W, Li X, et al. Cidea promotes hepatic steatosis by sensing dietary fatty acids. Hepatology. 2012;**56**(1):95-107

[43] Li JZ, Ye J, Xue B, Qi J, Zhang J, Zhou Z, et al. Cideb regulates diet-induced obesity, liver steatosis, and insulin sensitivity by controlling lipogenesis and fatty acid oxidation. Diabetes. 2007;**56**(10):2523-2532

[44] Li X, Ye J, Zhou L, Gu W, Fisher EA, Li P. Opposing roles of cell death-inducing DFF45-like effector B and perilipin 2 in controlling hepatic VLDL lipidation. Journal of Lipid Research. 2012;**53**(9):1877-1889

[45] Xu MJ, Cai Y, Wang H, Altamirano J, Chang B, Bertola A, et al. Fat-specific protein 27/CIDEC promotes development of alcoholic Steatohepatitis in mice and humans. Gastroenterology. 2015;**149**(4):1030-1041 e6

[46] Matsusue K, Kusakabe T, Noguchi T, Takiguchi S, Suzuki T, Yamano S, et al. Hepatic steatosis in leptin-deficient mice is promoted by the PPARgamma target gene Fsp27. Cell Metabolism. 2008;**7**(4):302-311

[47] Toh SY, Gong J, Du G, Li JZ, Yang S, Ye J, et al. Up-regulation of mitochondrial activity and acquirement of brown adipose tissue-like property in the white adipose tissue of fsp27 deficient mice. PLoS One. 2008;**3**(8):e2890

[48] Gong J, Sun Z, Wu L, Xu W, Schieber N, Xu D, et al. Fsp27 promotes lipid droplet growth by lipid exchange and transfer at lipid droplet contact sites. The Journal of Cell Biology. 2011;**195**(6):953-963

[49] Dollet L, Magre J, Cariou B, Prieur X. Function of seipin: New insights from Bscl2/seipin knockout mouse models. Biochimie. 2014;**96**:166-172

[50] Romeo S, Kozlitina J, Xing C, Pertsemlidis A, Cox D, Pennacchio LA, et al. Genetic variation in PNPLA3 confers susceptibility to nonalcoholic fatty liver disease. Nature Genetics. 2008;**40**(12):1461-1465

[51] Kitamoto T, Kitamoto A, Yoneda M, Hyogo H, Ochi H, Nakamura T, et al. Genome-wide scan revealed that polymorphisms in the PNPLA3, SAMM50, and PARVB genes are associated with development and progression of nonalcoholic fatty liver disease in Japan. Human Genetics. 2013;**132**(7):783-792

[52] He S, McPhaul C, Li JZ, Garuti R, Kinch L, Grishin NV, et al. A sequence variation (I148M) in PNPLA3 associated with nonalcoholic fatty liver disease disrupts triglyceride hydrolysis. The Journal of Biological Chemistry. 2010;**285**(9):6706-6715

[53] Pingitore P, Pirazzi C, Mancina RM, Motta BM, Indiveri C, Pujia A, et al. Recombinant PNPLA3 protein shows triglyceride hydrolase activity and its I148M mutation results in loss of function. Biochimica et Biophysica Acta. 2014;**1841**(4):574-580

[54] Pirazzi C, Valenti L, Motta BM, Pingitore P, Hedfalk K, Mancina RM, et al. PNPLA3 has retinyl-palmitate lipase activity in human hepatic stellate cells. Human Molecular Genetics. 2014;**23**(15):4077-4085

[55] Basantani MK, Sitnick MT, Cai L, Brenner DS, Gardner NP, Li JZ, et al. Pnpla3/Adiponutrin deficiency in mice does not contribute to fatty liver disease or metabolic syndrome. Journal of Lipid Research. 2011;**52**(2):318-329

[56] Chen W, Chang B, Li L, Chan L. Patatin-like phospholipase domain-containing 3/adiponutrin deficiency in mice is not associated with fatty liver disease. Hepatology. 2010;**52**(3):1134-1142

[57] Smagris E, BasuRay S, Li J, Huang Y, Lai KM, Gromada J, et al. Pnpla3I148M knockin mice accumulate PNPLA3 on lipid droplets and develop hepatic steatosis. Hepatology. 2015;**61**(1):108-118

[58] Pawella LM, Hashani M, Eiteneuer E, Renner M, Bartenschlager R, Schirmacher P, et al. Perilipin discerns chronic from acute hepatocellular steatosis. Journal of Hepatology. 2014;**60**(3):633-642

[59] Straub BK, Gyoengyoesi B, Koenig M, Hashani M, Pawella LM, Herpel E, et al. Adipophilin/perilipin-2 as a lipid droplet-specific marker for metabolically active cells and diseases associated with metabolic dysregulation. Histopathology. 2013;**62**(4):617-631

[60] Li H, Song Y, Zhang LJ, Gu Y, Li FF, Pan SY, et al. LSDP5 enhances triglyceride storage in hepatocytes by influencing lipolysis and fatty acid beta-oxidation of lipid droplets. PLoS One. 2012;**7**(6):e36712

[61] Beylot M, Neggazi S, Hamlat N, Langlois D, Forcheron F. Perilipin 1 ablation in mice enhances lipid oxidation during exercise and does not impair exercise performance. Metabolism. 2012;**61**(3):415-423

[62] Liu S, Geng B, Zou L, Wei S, Wang W, Deng J, et al. Development of hypertrophic cardiomyopathy in perilipin-1 null mice with adipose tissue dysfunction. Cardiovascular Research. 2015;**105**(1):20-30

[63] Varela GM, Antwi DA, Dhir R, Yin X, Singhal NS, Graham MJ, et al. Inhibition of ADRP prevents diet-induced insulin resistance. American Journal of Physiology. Gastrointestinal and Liver Physiology. 2008;**295**(3):G621-G628

[64] Imai Y, Varela GM, Jackson MB, Graham MJ, Crooke RM, Ahima RS. Reduction of hepatosteatosis and lipid levels by an adipose differentiation-related protein antisense oligonucleotide. Gastroenterology. 2007;**132**(5):1947-1954

[65] McManaman JL, Bales ES, Orlicky DJ, Jackman M, MacLean PS, Cain S, et al. Perilipin-2-null mice are protected against diet-induced obesity, adipose inflammation, and fatty liver disease. Journal of Lipid Research. 2013;**54**(5):1346-1359

[66] Carr RM, Peralta G, Yin X, Ahima RS. Absence of perilipin 2 prevents hepatic steatosis, glucose intolerance and ceramide accumulation in alcohol-fed mice. PLoS One. 2014;**9**(5):e97118

[67] Carr RM, Patel RT, Rao V, Dhir R, Graham MJ, Crooke RM, et al. Reduction of TIP47 improves hepatic steatosis and glucose homeostasis in mice. American Journal of Physiology. Regulatory, Integrative and Comparative Physiology. 2012;**302**(8):R996-1003

[68] Trevino MB, Mazur-Hart D, Machida Y, King T, Nadler J, Galkina EV, et al. Liver Perilipin 5 expression worsens Hepatosteatosis but not insulin resistance in high fat-fed mice. Molecular Endocrinology. 2015;**29**(10):1414-1425

[69] Haemmerle G, Lass A, Zimmermann R, Gorkiewicz G, Meyer C, Rozman J, et al. Defective lipolysis and altered energy metabolism in mice lacking adipose triglyceride lipase. Science. 2006;**312**(5774):734-737

[70] JW Wu, Wang SP, Alvarez F, Casavant S, Gauthier N, Abed L, et al. Deficiency of liver adipose triglyceride lipase in mice causes progressive hepatic steatosis. Hepatology. 2011;**54**(1):122-132

[71] Rasouli N, Molavi B, Elbein SC, Kern PA. Ectopic fat accumulation and metabolic syndrome. Diabetes, Obesity & Metabolism. 2007;**9**(1):1-10

[72] Boden G. Interaction between free fatty acids and glucose metabolism. Current Opinion in Clinical Nutrition and Metabolic Care. 2002;**5**(5):545-549

[73] Kovacs P, Stumvoll M. Fatty acids and insulin resistance in muscle and liver. Best Practice & Research. Clinical Endocrinology & Metabolism. 2005;**19**(4):625-635

[74] Minehira K, Young SG, Villanueva CJ, Yetukuri L, Oresic M, Hellerstein MK, et al. Blocking VLDL secretion causes hepatic steatosis but does not affect peripheral lipid stores or insulin sensitivity in mice. Journal of Lipid Research. 2008;**49**(9):2038-2044

[75] Petersen MC, Shulman GI. Roles of diacylglycerols and ceramides in hepatic insulin resistance. Trends in Pharmacological Sciences. 2017;**38**(7):649-665

[76] Cantley JL, Yoshimura T, Camporez JP, Zhang D, Jornayvaz FR, Kumashiro N, et al. CGI-58 knockdown sequesters diacylglycerols in lipid droplets/ER-preventing diacylglycerol-mediated hepatic insulin resistance. Proceedings of the National Academy of Sciences of the United States of America. 2013;**110**(5):1869-1874

[77] Samuel VT, Liu ZX, Wang A, Beddow SA, Geisler JG, Kahn M, et al. Inhibition of protein kinase Cepsilon prevents hepatic insulin resistance in nonalcoholic fatty liver disease. The Journal of Clinical Investigation. 2007;**117**(3):739-745

[78] Dries DR, Gallegos LL, Newton AC. A single residue in the C1 domain sensitizes novel protein kinase C isoforms to cellular diacylglycerol production. The Journal of Biological Chemistry. 2007;**282**(2):826-830

[79] Lipina C, Hundal HS. Sphingolipids: Agents provocateurs in the pathogenesis of insulin resistance. Diabetologia. 2011;**54**(7):1596-1607

[80] Singh R, Kaushik S, Wang Y, Xiang Y, Novak I, Komatsu M, et al. Autophagy regulates lipid metabolism. Nature. 2009;**458**(7242):1131-1135

[81] Tsai TH, Chen E, Li L, Saha P, Lee HJ, Huang LS, et al. The constitutive lipid droplet protein PLIN2 regulates autophagy in liver. Autophagy. 2017;**13**(7):1130-1144

[82] Rambold AS, Cohen S, Lippincott-Schwartz J. Fatty acid trafficking in starved cells: Regulation by lipid droplet lipolysis, autophagy, and mitochondrial fusion dynamics. Developmental Cell. 2015;**32**(6):678-692

[83] Shpilka T, Elazar Z. Lipid droplets regulate autophagosome biogenesis. Autophagy. 2015;**11**(11):2130-2131

[84] Shpilka T, Welter E, Borovsky N, Amar N, Mari M, Reggiori F, et al. Lipid droplets and their component triglycerides and steryl esters regulate autophagosome biogenesis. The EMBO Journal. 2015;**34**(16):2117-2131

[85] Yang L, Li P, Fu S, Calay ES, Hotamisligil GS. Defective hepatic autophagy in obesity promotes ER stress and causes insulin resistance. Cell Metabolism. 2010;**11**(6):467-478

[86] Ashraf NU, Sheikh TA. Endoplasmic reticulum stress and oxidative stress in the pathogenesis of non-alcoholic fatty liver disease. Free Radical Research. 2015;**49**(12):1405-1418

[87] Lee JS, Mendez R, Heng HH, Yang ZQ, Zhang K, Pharmacological ER. Stress promotes hepatic lipogenesis and lipid droplet formation. American Journal of Translational Research. 2012;**4**(1):102-113

[88] Fei W, Wang H, Fu X, Bielby C, Yang H. Conditions of endoplasmic reticulum stress stimulate lipid droplet formation in *Saccharomyces cerevisiae*. The Biochemical Journal. 2009;**424**(1):61-67

[89] Koek GH, Liedorp PR, Bast A. The role of oxidative stress in non-alcoholic steatohepatitis. Clinica Chimica Acta. 2011;**412**(15-16):1297-1305

[90] Videla LA, Rodrigo R, Orellana M, Fernandez V, Tapia G, Quinones L, et al. Oxidative stress-related parameters in the liver of non-alcoholic fatty liver disease patients. Clinical Science (London, England). 2004;**106**(3):261-268

[91] Videla LA, Rodrigo R, Araya J, Poniachik J. Insulin resistance and oxidative stress interdependency in non-alcoholic fatty liver disease. Trends in Molecular Medicine. 2006;**12**(12):555-558

[92] Hennig EE, Mikula M, Goryca K, Paziewska A, Ledwon J, Nesteruk M, et al. Extracellular matrix and cytochrome P450 gene expression can distinguish steatohepatitis from steatosis in mice. Journal of Cellular and Molecular Medicine. 2014;**18**(9):1762-1772

[93] Valenzuela R, Videla LA. The importance of the long-chain polyunsaturated fatty acid n-6/n-3 ratio in development of non-alcoholic fatty liver associated with obesity. Food & Function. 2011;**2**(11):644-648

[94] Videla LA, Rodrigo R, Araya J, Poniachik J. Oxidative stress and depletion of hepatic long-chain polyunsaturated fatty acids may contribute to nonalcoholic fatty liver disease. Free Radical Biology & Medicine. 2004;**37**(9):1499-1507

[95] Najt CP, Senthivinayagam S, Aljazi MB, Fader KA, Olenic SD, Brock JR, et al. Liver-specific loss of perilipin 2 alleviates diet-induced hepatic steatosis, inflammation, and fibrosis. American Journal of Physiology. Gastrointestinal and Liver Physiology. 2016;**310**(9):G726-G738

[96] Zheng P, Xie Z, Yuan Y, Sui W, Wang C, Gao X, et al. Plin5 alleviates myocardial ischaemia/reperfusion injury by reducing oxidative stress through inhibiting the lipolysis of lipid droplets. Scientific Reports. 2017;**7**:42574

[97] Zechner R, Kienesberger PC, Haemmerle G, Zimmermann R, Lass A. Adipose triglyceride lipase and the lipolytic catabolism of cellular fat stores. Journal of Lipid Research. 2009;**50**(1):3-21

[98] Yamaguchi T, Omatsu N, Morimoto E, Nakashima H, Ueno K, Tanaka T, et al. CGI-58 facilitates lipolysis on lipid droplets but is not involved in the vesiculation of lipid droplets caused by hormonal stimulation. Journal of Lipid Research. 2007;**48**(5):1078-1089

[99] Dalen KT, Ulven SM, Arntsen BM, Solaas K, Nebb HI. PPARalpha activators and fasting induce the expression of adipose differentiation-related protein in liver. Journal of Lipid Research. 2006;**47**(5):931-943

[100] Mishra R, Emancipator SN, Miller C, Kern T, Simonson MS. Adipose differentiation-related protein and regulators of lipid homeostasis identified by gene expression profiling in the murine db/db diabetic kidney. American Journal of Physiology. Renal Physiology. 2004;**286**(5):F913-F921

[101] Suzuki K, Takahashi K, Nishimaki-Mogami T, Kagechika H, Yamamoto M, Itabe H. Docosahexaenoic acid induces adipose differentiation-related protein through activation of retinoid x receptor in human choriocarcinoma BeWo cells. Biological & Pharmaceutical Bulletin. 2009;**32**(7):1177-1182

[102] Rankin EB, Rha J, Selak MA, Unger TL, Keith B, Liu Q, et al. Hypoxia-inducible factor 2 regulates hepatic lipid metabolism. Molecular and Cellular Biology. 2009;**29**(16):4527-4538

[103] Bindesboll C, Berg O, Arntsen B, Nebb HI, Dalen KT. Fatty acids regulate perilipin5 in muscle by activating PPARdelta. Journal of Lipid Research. 2013;**54**(7):1949-1963

[104] Granneman JG, Moore HP, Mottillo EP, Zhu Z. Functional interactions between Mldp (LSDP5) and Abhd5 in the control of intracellular lipid accumulation. The Journal of Biological Chemistry. 2009;**284**(5):3049-3057

[105] Huang Y, He S, Li JZ, Seo YK, Osborne TF, Cohen JC, et al. A feed-forward loop amplifies nutritional regulation of PNPLA3. Proceedings of the National Academy of Sciences of the United States of America. 2010;**107**(17):7892-7897

[106] Sathyanarayan A, Mashek MT, Mashek DG. ATGL promotes autophagy/lipophagy via SIRT1 to control hepatic lipid droplet catabolism. Cell Reports. 2017;**19**(1):1-9

[107] Cai H, Yao W, Li L, Li X, Hu L, Mai R, et al. Cell-death-inducing DFFA-like effector B contributes to the assembly of hepatitis C virus (HCV) particles and interacts with HCV NS5A. Scientific Reports. 2016;**6**:27778

[108] Chang BH, Li L, Saha P, Chan L. Absence of adipose differentiation related protein upregulates hepatic VLDL secretion, relieves hepatosteatosis, and improves whole body insulin resistance in leptin-deficient mice. Journal of Lipid Research. 2010;**51**(8):2132-2142

[109] Chang BH, Li L, Paul A, Taniguchi S, Nannegari V, Heird WC, et al. Protection against fatty liver but normal adipogenesis in mice lacking adipose differentiation-related protein. Molecular and Cellular Biology. 2006;**26**(3):1063-1076

[110] Zhou L, Park SY, Xu L, Xia X, Ye J, Su L, et al. Insulin resistance and white adipose tissue inflammation are uncoupled in energetically challenged Fsp27-deficient mice. Nature Communications. 2015;**6**:5949

[111] Langhi C, Arias N, Rajamoorthi A, Basta J, Lee RG, Baldan A. Therapeutic silencing of fat-specific protein 27 improves glycemic control in mouse models of obesity and insulin resistance. Journal of Lipid Research. 2017;**58**(1):81-91

[112] Liu L, Jiang Q, Wang X, Zhang Y, Lin RC, Lam SM, et al. Adipose-specific knockout of SEIPIN/BSCL2 results in progressive lipodystrophy. Diabetes. 2014;**63**(7):2320-2331

[113] Cui X, Wang Y, Meng L, Fei W, Deng J, Xu G, et al. Overexpression of a short human seipin/BSCL2 isoform in mouse adipose tissue results in mild lipodystrophy. American Journal of Physiology. Endocrinology and Metabolism. 2012;**302**(6):E705-E713

Nonalcoholic Fatty Liver Disease: The Future Frontier of Hepatology for South Asia

Shahinul Alam, Thupten Kelsang Lama,
Golam Mustafa, Mahabubul Alam and
Nooruddin Ahmad

Additional information is available at the end of the chapter

http://dx.doi.org/10.5772/intechopen.71159

Abstract

This review is to know the magnitude of nonalcoholic fatty liver disease (NAFLD) among general population and risk group populations of the South Asian countries. A thorough search of evidence-based literature was conducted using the PubMed database with key words. Databases searched from inception to February 2017. Systematic search of the literature was conducted for studies pertaining. Prevalence of NAFLD in South Asia varies from 13 to 34%. The Highest rate is in Bangladesh (34.34%) and lowest in Pakistan (13.5%). Prevalence of NAFLD is 15–80% among obese people, 25–60% with dyslipidemia and 33–55% in pre diabetics and diabetics. Nonalcoholic steatohepatitis (NASH) is present in about 50% of the NAFLD cases that can lead to fibrosis, cirrhosis or even hepatocellular carcinoma (HCC). NAFLD is not the disease for only obese people, but it is also common in nonobese in this region. About 11.11% hepatocellular carcinoma developed from NASH. Incidence rate of diabetes and coronary artery disease is high among NAFLD patients. NAFLD is becoming a future challenge for South Asia region. Prevalence and severity has been remarkably increasing for last few years. The health system should get ready to confront burden of NAFLD in future for South Asia.

Keywords: nonalcoholic fatty liver disease, nonalcoholic steatohepatitis, South Asia

1. Introduction

Nonalcoholic fatty liver disease (NAFLD) is a characterized by excessive accumulation of fat (defined as the presence of lipid in >5% of hepatocytes or a lipid content >5% of liver weight) [1] in the liver, who consume little (<20 g of alcohol/d) or no alcohol [1, 2]. It is the most common cause of chronic liver injury [3]. Worldwide millions of people are affected by the NAFLD and it is prophesied to be the following universal epidemic [4]. Universally its prevalence rate is 25.24 with highest in the Middle East and South America and lowest in Africa [5]. The NAFLD with necroinflammation, defined as nonalcoholic steatohepatitis (NASH) [2]. According to Younossi ZM, universally overall mortality for NAFLD is 1.05; and incidence of hepatocellular carcinoma (HCC) and liver-specific mortality among NAFLD is 0.44 and 0.77 per 1000 person-years respectively. About 30% NAFLD progress to NASH, it can be lead to fibrosis, cirrhosis or even hepatocellular carcinoma [6]. HCC is one of the most common cancers worldwide and its burden is highest in the South-East Asia [7]. Countries with higher economic status tend to present a higher prevalence of NAFLD [8]. But it is not uncommon in low economic countries like countries of South Asia. The prevalence of NAFLD has increased remarkably over the years in South Asia and South-East Asia affecting 5–34% of general population [9, 10]. Metabolic syndrome common in people from South Asia is an important risk factor for NAFLD and Bangladeshi ethnicity is an important independent risk factor for NAFLD [3]. It is commonly described as hepatic manifestation of metabolic syndrome and insulin resistance. Though prevalence of NAFLD markedly increased in obese population, presence of NAFLD is further more challenging to diagnose and manage in lean population. In this study we aimed to know the prevalence NAFLD among general population and risk group populations of the South Asian countries. We also explored the prevalence of NASH and its associated conditions.

2. Materials and methods

We performed a systematic PubMed/MEDLINE literature search with the following key words: "Non-alcoholic Fatty Liver Disease/epidemiology"[Mesh], "Non-alcoholic steatohepatitis" [Text word] AND "Liver Transplantation/etiology"[Mesh], "Obesity"[Mesh], "Diabetes Mellitus"[Mesh], "Global," "Afghanistan," "Pakistan," "India," "Sri Lanka," "Maldives," "Nepal," "Bangladesh," and "Bhutan." Databases searched from inception to February 2017. Exclusions included data on alcohol consumption or other liver diseases. Relevant full article, abstract, review, mini review, editorial and conference proceeding are included in this review.

3. Global epidemiology

Nonalcoholic fatty liver disease (NAFLD) is the commonest liver disease with global prevalence of approximately 25.24% of the general population [5]. Nonalcoholic steatohepatitis (NASH) and NAFLD are not only a Western disease. NAFLD and NASH have increasingly been diagnosed in all regions of Asia [11]. A study using the National Health and Nutrition Examination Survey (NHANES) found a 30% prevalence of NAFLD in the United States between 2011 and 2012 [12]. NAFLD is the most common cause of chronic liver disease in Western countries. It affects about 1 billion individuals worldwide [13]. Increasing prevalence of NASH is closely associated with prevalence diabetes and obesity, which may defined as epidemic worldwide. At least 1.46 billion obese adult is persisting in the world. Approximately 6 million individuals in the USA are in the risk of developing NASH and about 0.6 million

Region	Population studied	Prevalence of NAFLD in these populations (%)
USA	Pediatric population	13–14
	General population	27–34
Europe	Pediatric population	2.6–10
	General population	20–30
Middle East	General population	20–30
Far East	General population	15
South Asia	General population	5–30

Table 1. Estimated prevalence of NAFLD and NASH among different areas of the word.

to develop NASH-related cirrhosis [14]. **Table 1** shows estimated prevalence of NAFLD and NASH. Reports on the prevalence of NAFLD and NASH vary substantially due to varying definitions, differences in the populations studied, and the diagnostic methods used [14].

4. Delineation of South Asia and its population diversity

According to the United Nations geographic region ordering, South Asia comprised with Afghanistan, Bangladesh, Bhutan, India, Maldives, Nepal, Pakistan, and Sri Lanka (**Figure 1**). Topographically, it is dominated by the Indian Plate; the terms "Indian subcontinent" and "South Asia" are sometimes used interchangeably [15]. South Asia is the most populated region in the world [16]. Socially it is very mixed, consisting of many language groups and religions, and social practices in one region that are vastly different from those in another [17].

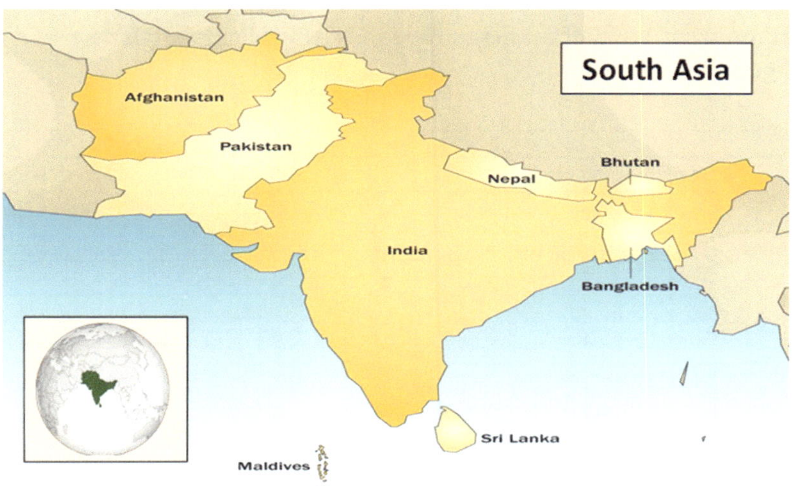

Figure 1. Geographical position and area of South Asia [16].

5. Prevalence of NAFLD among South Asian people

Recent socioeconomic changes have resulted in an emerging epidemic of non-communicable diseases such as type 2 diabetes and nonalcoholic fatty liver disease. The prevalence of nonalcoholic fatty liver disease in Asian Pacific countries now approximates and even overrides levels encountered in Western countries in some studies [18]. NAFLD is the emerging challenge for public health issue in Asia [19]. This has a potential burden not only on liver disease but also on metabolic syndrome related morbidity: obesity, diabetes, and atherosclerotic cardiovascular disease [19]. Largest population of the world inhabiting in Asia are passing through an economic growth and shift of focus from a dominant physical activity to knowledge, capital and physical inactivity. An increasing GDP is paralleled by a rising body mass index (BMI) in an almost linear fashion [19]. Countries with higher economic status tend to present a higher prevalence of NAFLD [8]. It is believed to provide a distinctive epidemiologic perspective to global situation of NAFLD. Especially for South Asia, according to increasing with their economy the prevalence of NAFLD is increasing day by day.

Most of the available epidemiological studies in NAFLD from Asia are ultrasound based and hence detect prevalence of hepatic steatosis alone initially, correlating it with anthropometric, biochemical, and demographic features of the population (**Table 2**). The community prevalence of NAFLD in South Asia and South-East Asia ranges from 5 to 30% [9, 10]. Recently a hospital based study in Pakistan had shown a frequency of approximately 14%. In India, it varies from 5 to 28% in general population, especially those who are undergoing health check-ups. Indians have increased propensity for visceral fat accumulation which may present from birth [9]. Prevalence of NAFLD in general population of Bangladesh has been estimated to vary from 4 to 34.34% [20, 21], which exceeds previous reports and it jumps up to 49.8% in diabetic patients [22, 23]. And in Sri Lanka the prevalence rate was found 32.6 in an urban based study [24]. So it is seen that, among South Asian countries the highest magnitude of NAFLD is in Bangladesh and lowest is in Pakistan (**Figure 2**).

Country	Population and place	Sample size (*n*)	Prevalence of NAFL
India	Selected population Mumbai	1168	16.6%
	General population West Bengal (rural)	1911	167 (8.7%)
	General population Chennai (urban)	541	173 (32%)
Bangladesh	General population Nation wide	2621	900 (34.34%)
	Selected Population Camilla (rural)	665	219 (33%)
Sri Lanka	General population (urban)	2985	974 (32.6%)
Pakistan	Tertiary care hospital, Karachi	952	129 (13.5%)

Table 2. Prevalence of NAFLD among the Indian, Sri Lanka and Pakistani people.

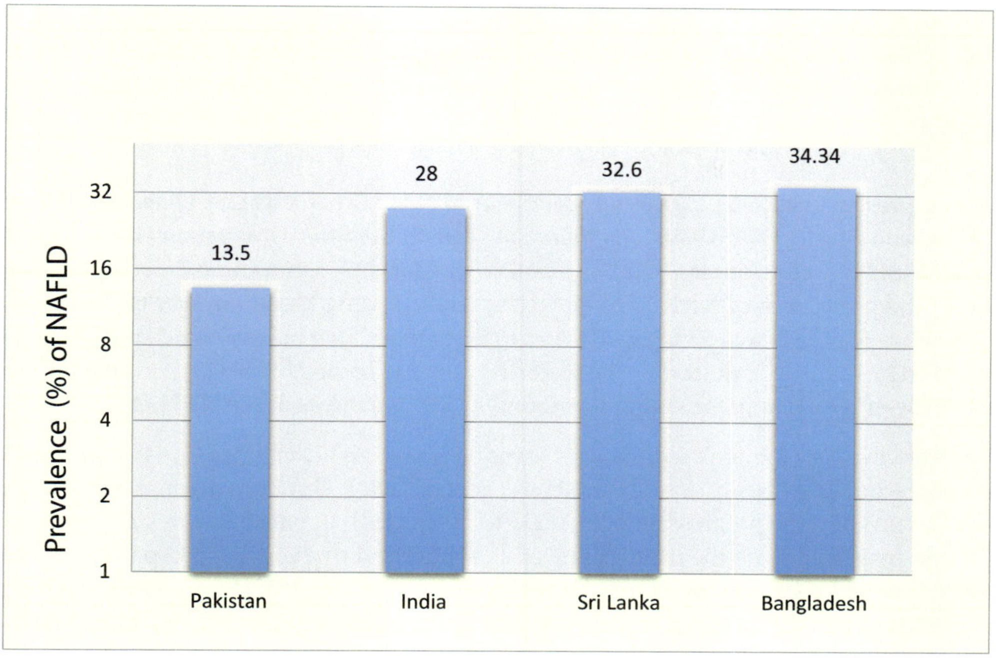

Figure 2. Prevalence of NAFLD in different countries of South Asia.

From the study of Alazawi et al. the prevalence of recorded NAFLD varied considerably by ethnic group. This study identified that Bangladeshi ethnicity as an independent risk factor for NAFLD. Diagnosed NAFLD was significantly more prevalent among people of Bangladesh ethnicity (1.8% of the adult population) than other ethnic group, including other South Asian groups. Among Bangladeshis, there are higher rates of type 2 diabetes and cardiovascular disease that may have a genetic basis. Transaminase were measured on 218,032 patients, of whom 31,627 had elevated serum transaminases. In a multivariate analysis, independent risk factors for NAFLD included Bangladeshi ethnicity, diabetes, raised BMI, hypertension, and hypercholesterolaemia. As expected, the prevalence of NAFLD was significantly lower in the African and Caribbean ethnic groups [19]. Female are predominant sufferers of NAFLD in Bangladesh [25]. So the prevalence of NAFLD in South Asia has been increased from previous reports and now it ranges from 14 to 34.34% in general population. In systematic searching in PubMed/MEDLINE database, we found research articles on epidemiology of NAFLD of India, Bangladesh, Sri Lanka and Pakistan. But we did not get any article relevant to the epidemiology of NAFLD of Afghanistan, Maldives, Nepal and Bhutan.

6. Prevalence of NASH and its progression

The active form of NAFLD is non-alcoholic steatohepatitis (NASH), which is characterized by hepatocyte injury with liver inflammation, and progression of fibrosis [26]. And it has emerged as one of the most important causes of liver failure and hepatocellular carcinoma. Up to 20% of cases NASH may progress to cirrhosis [27]. According to Alam et al. "Patients with NASH are at risk for progressive liver disease (which can progress to cirrhosis, hepatocellular carcinoma, and death from chronic liver disease), as well as cardiovascular mortality and type-2 diabetes" [25].

NASH is present in 42.4–53.1% cases of Bangladeshi NAFLD patients [25]. Diabetic is the principle cause to develop NASH. A study in Indian Diabetic Mellitus (DM) patient; it reported that severe NASH is present among 9.35% Indian DM patients [28]. Ultrasound based Indian study showed the prevalence of NAFLD to be 16.6%, while a study based on liver biopsy showed the presence of NASH was 53% [29, 30]. And in Sri Lanka a liver biopsy based study were performed on 296 patients and 100 (35.1%) were diagnosed as having NASH [31]. In another Asian study proven NASH at presentation was found in 32.6% patients of NAFLD [32].

Study from the West found that disease progression from NAFLD to NASH is 44% patients [33]. Multiple factors like obesity, insulin resistance, genetic factor, immune response and lipotoxicity are involved in the progression of NAFLD to NASH [34]. In patients with cirrhotic NASH, HCC and liver failure are the main causes of morbidity and mortality. A prospective Japanese study elucidated the progression from NASH to HCC is 11.3% [35]. The prevalence of NASH (9.35–59%) among NAFLD patients is much higher in South Asian countries than that of Western countries. Severity of NAFLD in the form of NASH is also highest in Bangladesh among the South Asian countries as evidenced by recent studies from tertiary level hospitals of the country.

7. Depiction of the magnitude among different risk group

According to Alam, one fourth of the Bangladeshi NAFLD patients are nonobese; among them 53.1% cases present NASH. Male are largely dominating in nonobese group, where female are in obese group [36]. High BMI, central obesity, triglyceridemia and age are important risk factors for Bangladeshi people, and risk factors contributed about 29% risk for the occurrence of NASH [37]. After adjusting the risk factors (BMI and TG) female gender is the independent risk for Bangladeshi [38]. Although insulin resistance (IR) is strongly associated with NAFLD, But IR is not the sole predictor in the pathogenesis of NAFLD [38–40].

In India the prevalence of NAFLD is 15–80% among obese people, 25–60% in patients with dyslipidemia and 33–55% in pre-diabetics and diabetics' Indian people [41]. Most of the non-diabetic NAFLD patients are overweight/obese with higher insulin resistance, dyslipidemia, and subclinical inflammation [42]. Among 65.7% Morbidly Obese South Indian Patients has NAFLD. Among them 33.6% were of NASH, 31.3% shows fibrosis and 14.1% shows advanced fibrosis [43]. The polymorphism T-455C in APOC3 gene and elevated serum triglycerides are associated with Indian NAFLD patients [44]. In another series, 56.5% T2DM patients have NAFLD, and the prevalence is higher in females (60%) than males T2DM patients [45]. NAFLD is the commonest liver disease in Indian psoriatic patients also [46]. Coronary artery disease (CAD) is more prevalent in the NAFLD compared to non-NAFLD; It is a surrogate

http://dx.doi.org/10.5772/intechopen.71159

and fairly reliable marker of risk for CAD among type 2 diabetic patients [47]. According to Duseja NAFLD is the commonest cause of unexplained elevation of SGPT and cryptogenic cirrhosis and hepatocellular carcinoma in Indian patients. Insulin resistance and full blown metabolic syndrome are highly prevalent in Indian patients with NAFLD [48]; 51.4% of patients of NAFLD have metabolic syndrome [49]. And it is really threatening news that 3% of 5–12 years Indian children have NAFLD [50].

In Sri Lanka Incidence rate of diabetes are 64.2 per 1000 person-years among NAFLD persons [51]. NAFLD is an independent predictor of developing diabetes mellitus [51]. Increased age and presence of NAFLD conferred a higher mortality risk from ACS as predicted by GRACE score [52].

As like developed countries obesity, insulin resistance, diabetes, dyslipidemia are the major risk factors for development of NAFLD. But the paradox is that it could develop in nonobese population also and one fourth of NAFLD of South Asia is from nonobese people.

8. Global and South Asian publication trend on NAFLD

According to Zhang et al. study, with the globally increasing prevalence, nonalcoholic fatty liver disease (NAFLD) becomes the predominant cause of chronic liver disease. The global scientific research articles relevant to NAFLD revealed 6356 articles were published in 994 different journals during 1986–2013. Starting from the late 1980s, the publication on NAFLD grew slowly and entered into a highly developing period in the 21st century, especially in the last decade (**Figure 3**). Bibliometric results suggest that the obviously rapid growth of the

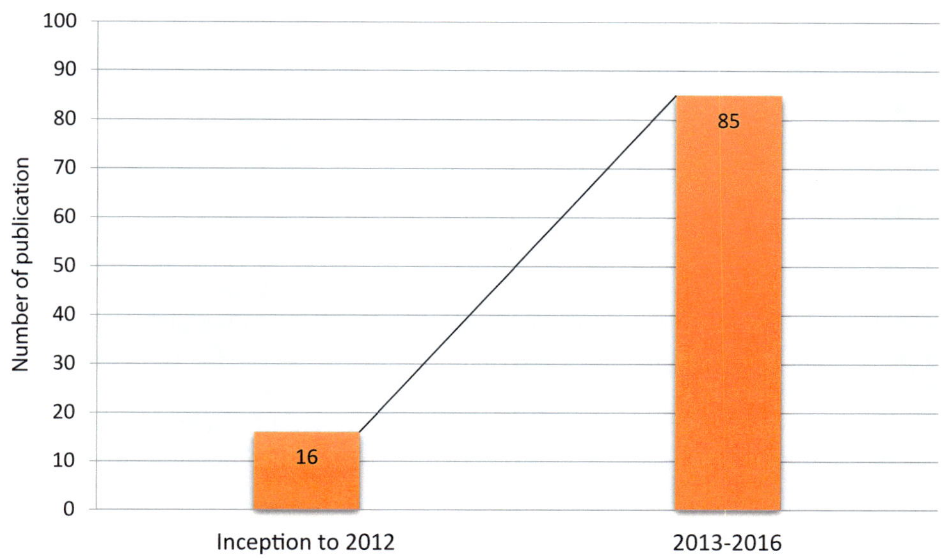

Figure 3. Trend of number of publication on NAFLD of South Asia (published in PubMed).

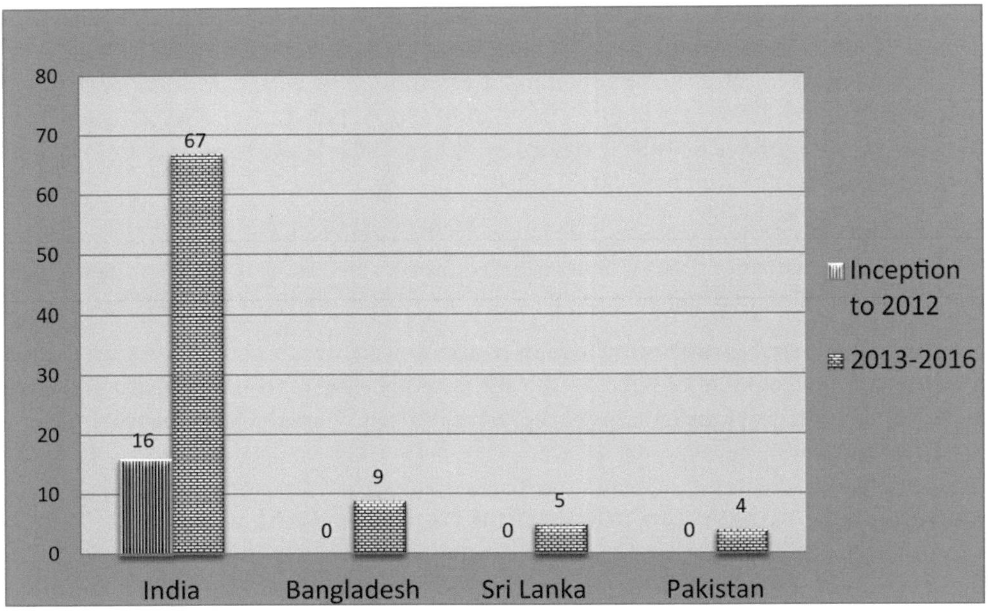

Figure 4. Article on NAFLD publication in South Asia Trend in PubMed from inception-2016.

articles in recent years appears to be associated with the accelerating incidence of NAFLD and its cofactors such as metabolic syndrome. In this study we found that, from inception to 2012 only 16 Indian research articles have been published in PubMed. Where from 2013 to 2016 total 85 research articles of India, Bangladesh, Sri Lanka and Pakistan has been published in PubMed (**Figure 4**). This phenomenon indicate that, how NAFLD is growing in South Asia.

9. Conclusion

The increase in NAFLD will continue to burden the health care system, especially because of its association with obesity, IR and metabolic syndrome. Along with globalization the prevalence of NAFLD is increasing alarmingly. The prevalence of NAFLD has been increasing remarkably for the last 12 years. Currently it is not only a disease of the Western countries but also becoming a major challenge for South Asia region. NAFLD is not the disease for only obese people, but it is also common in nonobese. And if the condition remains untreated it can turn into cirrhosis and hepatocellular carcinoma. It is really a great threat for us that, NAFLD is being seeing among our subcontinent's children also. The burden of NAFLD and its severity projects that obviously it will be the biggest frontier of Hepatology in South Asia in near future.

Author details

Shahinul Alam[1]*, Thupten Kelsang Lama[2], Golam Mustafa[1], Mahabubul Alam[1] and Nooruddin Ahmad[1]

Address all correspondence to: shahinul67@yahoo.com

1 Department of Hepatology, Bangabandhu Sheikh Mujib Medical University, Dhaka, Bangladesh

2 Civil Service Hospital, Kathmandu, Nepal

References

[1] Arab JP, Candia R, Zapata R, Munoz C, Arancibia JP, Poniachik J, Soza A, Fuster F, Brahm J, Sanhueza E, Contreras J, Cuellar MC, Arrese M, Riquelme A. Management of nonalcoholic fatty liver disease: An evidence-based clinical practice review. World Journal of Gastroenterology. 2014;**20**:12182-12201 [PMID: 25232252]. DOI: 10.3748/wjg.v20.i34.12182

[2] Zhang TS, Qin HL, Wang T, Li HT, Li H, Xia SH, Xiang XH. Global publication trends and research hotspots of nonalcoholic fatty liver disease: A bibliometric analysis and systematic review. SpringerPlus. 2015;**4**:776 [PMID: 26697286]. DOI: 10.1186/s40064-015-1542-1

[3] Alazawi W, Mathur R, Abeysekera K, Hull S, Boomla K, Robson J, Foster GR. Ethnicity and the diagnosis gap in liver disease: A population-based study. The British Journal of General Practice. 2014;**64**:e694-e702 [PMID: 25348993]. DOI: 10.3399/bjgp14X682273

[4] Sherif ZA, Saeed A, Ghavimi S, Nouraie SM, Laiyemo AO, Brim H, Ashktorab H. Global epidemiology of nonalcoholic fatty liver disease and perspectives on US Minority populations. Digestive Diseases and Sciences. 2016;**61**:1214-1225 [PMID: 27038448]. DOI: 10.1007/s10620-016-4143-0

[5] Younossi ZM, Koenig AB, Abdelatif D, Fazel Y, Henry L, Wymer M. Global epidemiology of nonalcoholic fatty liver disease-meta-analytic assessment of prevalence, incidence, and outcomes. Hepatology. 2016;**64**:73-84. [PMID: 26707365]. DOI: 10.1002/hep.28431

[6] Chalasani N, Younossi Z, Lavine JE, Diehl AM, Brunt EM, Cusi K, Charlton M, Sanyal AJ. The diagnosis and management of non-alcoholic fatty liver disease: Practice Guideline by the American Association for the Study of Liver Diseases, American College of Gastroenterology, and the American Gastroenterological Association. Hepatology. 2012;**55**:2005-2023 [PMID: 22488764]. DOI: 10.1002/hep.25762

[7] Ashtari S, Pourhoseingholi MA, Zali MR. Non-alcohol fatty liver disease in Asia: Prevention and planning. World Journal of Hepatology. 2015;**7**:1788-1796 [PMID: 26167252]. DOI: 10.4254/wjh.v7.i13.1788

[8] Zhu JZ, Dai YN, Wang YM, Zhou QY, CH Y, Li YM. Prevalence of nonalcoholic fatty liver disease and economy. Digestive Diseases and Sciences. 2015;**60**:3194-3202. [PMID: 26017679]. DOI: 10.1007/s10620-015-3728-3

[9] Parkash O, Hamid S. Are we ready for a new epidemic of under recognized liver disease in South Asia especially in Pakistan? Nonalcoholic fatty liver disease. The Journal of the Pakistan Medical Association. 2013;**63**:95-99 [PMID: 23865141]

[10] Chan WK, Tan AT, Vethakkan SR, Tah PC, Vijayananthan A, Goh KL. Low physical activity and energy dense Malaysian foods are associated with non-alcoholic fatty liver disease in centrally obese but not in non-centrally obese patients with diabetes mellitus. Asia Pacific Journal of Clinical Nutrition. 2015;**24**:289-298 [PMID: 26078246]. DOI: 10.6133/apjcn.2015.24.2.15

[11] Rahman MM, Abedin T, Amin R, Rahman MR, Faiz MA. Nonalcoholic fatty liver disease—Is it always benign? Journal of Bangladesh College of Physicians and Surgeons. 2007;**25**(3):144-152. DOI: 10.3329/jbcps.v25i3.411

[12] Ruhl CE, Everhart JE. Fatty liver indices in the multiethnic United States National Health and Nutrition Examination Survey. Alimentary Pharmacology & Therapeutics. 2015;**41**:65-76 [PMID: 25376360]. DOI: 10.1111/apt.13012

[13] Munteanu MA, Nagy GA, Mircea PA. Current management of NAFLD. Clujul Medical. 2016;**89**:19-23. [PMID: 27004021]. DOI: 10.15386/cjmed-539

[14] LaBrecque DR, Abbas Z, Anania F, Ferenci P, Khan AG, Goh KL, Hamid SS, Isakov V, Lizarzabal M, Penaranda MM, Ramos JF, Sarin S, Stimac D, Thomson AB, Umar M, Krabshuis J, LeMair A. World Gastroenterology Organisation global guidelines: Nonalcoholic fatty liver disease and nonalcoholic steatohepatitis. Journal of Clinical Gastroenterology. 2014;**48**:467-473. [PMID: 24921212]. DOI: 10.1097/mcg.0000000000000116

[15] Pandit K, Goswami S, Ghosh S, Mukhopadhyay P, Chowdhury S. Metabolic syndrome in South Asians. Indian Journal of Endocrinology and Metabolism. 2012;**16**:44-55. [PMID: 22276252]. DOI: 10.4103/2230-8210.91187

[16] United Nations, Department of Economic and Social Affairs, Population Division. World Urbanization Prospects: The 2014 Revision. The United Nations, New York; 2014

[17] Baten J. A History of the Global Economy. Cambridge, UK: Cambridge University Press; 2016

[18] Mahady SE, George J. The future liver of the Asia pacific: Fatter and firmer from more fructose and fortune? Journal of Clinical and Experimental Hepatology. 2013;**3**:106-113 [PMID: 25755484]. DOI: 10.1016/j.jceh.2012.10.011

[19] Chowdhury A, Younossi ZM. Global epidemiology and risk factors for nonalcoholic fatty liver disease. Alcoholic and Non-Alcoholic Fatty Liver Disease: Springer. 2016:21-40

[20] Alam S, Chowdhury MAB, Azam G, Ahsan M, Mustafa G, Hossain M, Khan M, Ahmed N. Prevalence of fatty liver in Bangladesh: A nation wide population based study. Hepatology International. 2017;**11**:S553. DOI: 10.1007/s12072-016-9783-9

[21] Hoque MK, AMM, Islam MB. Prevalence of non-alcoholic fatty liver disease in rural population of Bangladesh. Hepatology International. 2017;**11**:S961. DOI: 10.1007/s12072-016-9783-9

[22] Hoque MI. NAFLD in Bangladesh. Abstract Book 1st Conference of SASL2013. p. 69

[23] Rahman MMKM, Begum H, Haque M, Sultana N, Akhter M. Prevalence and risk factors of nonalcoholic fatty liver disease in a rural Community of South Asia. Gastroenterology Research and Practice. 2015;**148**:S1045-S1046

[24] Dassanayake AS, Kasturiratne A, Rajindrajith S, Kalubowila U, Chakrawarthi S, De Silva AP, Makaya M, Mizoue T, Kato N, Wickremasinghe AR, de Silva HJ. Prevalence and risk factors for non-alcoholic fatty liver disease among adults in an urban Sri Lankan population. Journal of Gastroenterology and Hepatology. 2009;**24**:1284-1288 [PMID: 19476560. DOI: 10.1111/j.1440-1746.2009.05831.x

[25] Alam S, Noor EASM, Chowdhury ZR, Alam M, Kabir J. Nonalcoholic steatohepatitis in nonalcoholic fatty liver disease patients of Bangladesh. World Journal of Hepatology. 2013;**5**:281-287 [PMID: 23717739]. DOI: 10.4254/wjh.v5.i5.281

[26] Wong VW-S, Chitturi S, Wong GL-H, Yu J, Chan HL-Y, Farrell GC. Pathogenesis and novel treatment options for non-alcoholic steatohepatitis. The Lancet Gastroenterology & Hepatology. 2016;**1**:56-67

[27] Matteoni CA, Younossi ZM, Gramlich T, Boparai N, Liu YC, McCullough AJ. Nonalcoholic fatty liver disease: A spectrum of clinical and pathological severity. Gastroenterology. 1999;**116**(6):1413-1419 [PMID: 10348825]

[28] Gupte P, Amarapurkar D, Agal S, Baijal R, Kulshrestha P, Pramanik S, Patel N, Madan A, Amarapurkar A. Non-alcoholic steatohepatitis in type 2 diabetes mellitus. Journal of Gastroenterology and Hepatology. 2004;**19**:854-858

[29] Yilmaz Y, Eren F. A Bayesian approach to an integrated multimodal noninvasive diagnosis of definitive nonalcoholic steatohepatitis in the spectrum of nonalcoholic fatty liver disease. European Journal of Gastroenterology & Hepatology. 2014;**26**:1292-1295 [PMID: 25171027]. DOI: 10.1097/meg.0000000000000184

[30] Duseja A, Das A, Das R, Dhiman RK, Chawla Y, Bhansali A, Kalra N. The clinicopathological profile of Indian patients with nonalcoholic fatty liver disease (NAFLD) is different from that in the West. Digestive Diseases and Sciences. 2007;**52**:2368-2374 [PMID: 17420951]. DOI: 10.1007/s10620-006-9136-y

[31] De Hewavisenthi SJ, Dassanayaka AS, De Silva HJ. Clinical, biochemical and histological characteristics of a Sri Lankan population of non-alcoholic steatohepatitis (NASH) patients. The Ceylon Medical Journal. 2005;**50**:113-116 [PMID: 16252575]

[32] Wong VW, Wong GL, Choi PC, Chan AW, Li MK, Chan HY, Chim AM, Yu J, Sung JJ, Chan HL. Disease progression of non-alcoholic fatty liver disease: A prospective study with paired liver biopsies at 3 years. Gut. 2010;**59**:969-974. [PMID: 20581244]. DOI: 10.1136/gut.2009.205088

[33] McPherson S, Hardy T, Henderson E, Burt AD, Day CP, Anstee QM. Evidence of NAFLD progression from steatosis to fibrosing-steatohepatitis using paired biopsies: Implications for prognosis and clinical management. Journal of Hepatology. 2015;**62**:1148-1155 [PMID: 25477264]. DOI: 10.1016/j.jhep.2014.11.034

[34] Sharma M, Mitnala S, Vishnubhotla RK, Mukherjee R, Reddy DN, Rao PN. The riddle of nonalcoholic fatty liver disease: Progression from nonalcoholic fatty liver to nonalcoholic steatohepatitis. Journal of Clinical and Experimental Hepatology. 2015;**5**:147-158 [PMID: 26155043]. DOI: 10.1016/j.jceh.2015.02.002

[35] Hashimoto E, Tokushige K. Prevalence, gender, ethnic variations, and prognosis of NASH. Journal of Gastroenterology. 2011;**46**:S63-S69 [PMID: 20844903]. DOI: 10.1007/s00535-010-0311-8

[36] Alam S, Gupta UD, Alam M, Kabir J, Chowdhury ZR, Alam AK. Clinical, anthropometric, biochemical, and histological characteristics of nonobese nonalcoholic fatty liver disease patients of Bangladesh. Indian Journal of Gastroenterology. 2014;**33**:452-457 [PMID: 25023045]. DOI: 10.1007/s12664-014-0488-5

[37] Majid N, Ali Z, Rahman MR, Akhter A, Rajib RC, Ahmad F, Sharmin S, Akond AK, Huq N. Histological scoring and associated risk factors of non-alcoholic fatty liver disease. Mymensingh Medical Journal. 2013;**22**:767-772 [PMID: 24292310]

[38] Hossain IA, Akter S, Rahman MK, Ali L. Gender specific association of serum leptin and insulinemic indices with nonalcoholic fatty liver disease in prediabetic subjects. PLoS One. 2015;**10**:e0142165 [PMID: 26569494]. DOI: 10.1371/journal.pone.0142165

[39] Alam S, Mustafa G, Alam M, Ahmad N. Insulin resistance in development and progression of nonalcoholic fatty liver disease. World Journal of Gastrointestinal Pathophysiology. 2016;**7**:211-217 [PMID: 27190693]. DOI: 10.4291/wjgp.v7.i2.211

[40] Hossain IA, Rahman Shah MM, Rahman MK, Ali L. Gamma glutamyl transferase is an independent determinant for the association of insulin resistance with nonalcoholic fatty liver disease in Bangladeshi adults: Association of GGT and HOMA-IR with NAFLD. Diabetes and Metabolic Syndrome: Clinical Research and Reviews. 2016;**10**:S25-S29. [PMID: 26482965]. DOI: 10.1016/j.dsx.2015.09.005

[41] Tandon RK. Emergence of non-alcoholic fatty liver disease (NAFLD). Journal of the Association of Physicians of India. 2013;**61**:445-446 [PMID: 24772745]

[42] Bhatt SP, Misra A, Nigam P, Guleria R, Pasha MA. Phenotype, body composition, and prediction equations (Indian fatty liver index) for non-alcoholic fatty liver disease in non-diabetic Asian Indians: A case-control study. PLoS One. 2015;**10**:e0142260 [PMID: 26599361]. DOI: 10.1371/journal.pone.0142260

[43] Praveenraj P, Gomes RM, Kumar S, Karthikeyan P, Shankar A, Parthasarathi R, Senthilnathan P, Rajapandian S, Palanivelu C. Prevalence and predictors of non-alcoholic fatty liver disease in morbidly obese south indian patients undergoing bariatric surgery. Obesity Surgery. 2015;**25**:2078-2087 [PMID: 25835982]. DOI: 10.1007/s11695-015-1655-1

[44] Puppala J, Bhrugumalla S, Kumar A, Siddapuram SP, Viswa PD, Kondawar M, Akka J, Munshi A. Apolipoprotein C3 gene polymorphisms in Southern Indian patients with nonalcoholic fatty liver disease. Indian Journal of Gastroenterology. 2014;**33**:524-529 [PMID: 25319715]. DOI: 10.1007/s12664-014-0504-9

[45] Kalra S, Vithalani M, Gulati G, Kulkarni CM, Kadam Y, Pallivathukkal J, Das B, Sahay R, Modi KD. Study of prevalence of nonalcoholic fatty liver disease (NAFLD) in type 2 diabetes patients in India (SPRINT). The Journal of the Association of Physicians of India. 2013;**61**:448-453 [PMID: 24772746]

[46] Madanagobalane S, Anandan S. The increased prevalence of non-alcoholic fatty liver disease in psoriatic patients: A study from South India. Australian Journal of Dermatology. 2012;**53**:190-197 [PMID: 22672067]. DOI: 10.1111/j.1440-0960.2012.00905.x

[47] Agarwal AK, Jain V, Singla S, Baruah BP, Arya V, Yadav R, Singh VP. Prevalence of non-alcoholic fatty liver disease and its correlation with coronary risk factors in patients with type 2 diabetes. The Journal of the Association of Physicians of India. 2011;**59**:351-354 [PMID: 21751587]

[48] Duseja A. Nonalcoholic fatty liver disease in India—A lot done, yet more required! Indian Journal of Gastroenterology. 2010;**29**:217-225 [PMID: 21191681]. DOI: 10.1007/s12664-010-0069-1

[49] Gaharwar R, Trikha S, Margekar SL, Jatav OP, Ganga PD. Study of clinical profile of patients of nonalcoholic fatty liver disease and its association with metabolic syndrome. The Journal of the Association of Physicians of India. 2015;**63**:12-16 [PMID: 26591121]

[50] Chaturvedi K, Vohra P. Non-alcoholic fatty liver disease in children. Indian Pediatrics. 2012;**49**:757-758 [PMID: 23024085]

[51] Kasturiratne A, Weerasinghe S, Dassanayake AS, Rajindrajith S, de Silva AP, Kato N, Wickremasinghe AR, de Silva HJ. Influence of non-alcoholic fatty liver disease on the development of diabetes mellitus. Journal of Gastroenterology and Hepatology. 2013;**28**:142-147 [PMID: 22989165]. DOI: 10.1111/j.1440-1746.2012.07264.x

[52] Perera N, Indrakumar J, Abeysinghe WV, Fernando V, Samaraweera W, Lawrence JS. Nonalcoholic fatty liver disease increases the mortality from acute coronary syndrome: An observational study from Sri Lanka. BMC Cardiovascular Disorders. 2016;**16**:1

Chapter 5

Noninvasive Evaluation of Fibrosis and Steatosis in Nonalcoholic Fatty Liver Disease by Elastographic Methods

Monica Lupsor-Platon

Additional information is available at the end of the chapter

http://dx.doi.org/10.5772/intechopen.71161

Abstract

An increasingly common cause of chronic liver disease in adults and children is nonalcoholic fatty liver disease (NAFLD). The diagnosis of NAFLD was traditionally based on the histopathological changes of the liver, evaluated by needle liver biopsy, an invasive method, with potential adverse effects and great inter and intraobserver variability. The noninvasive methods for the assessment of both fibrosis and steatosis in patients with NAFLD have increasingly been studied lately. Of these noninvasive methods, in this chapter, we will focus on the methods assessing the stiffness of liver parenchyma, i.e. elastographic methods, of which, the most widely used are ultrasound elastography techniques. We will discuss the principal elastographic methods of some utility in NAFLD, i.e. shear wdave elastography (SWE) (quantitative elastography), and especially transient elastography, point SWE (acoustic radiation force impulse elastography, ARFI) and two-dimensional real-time SWE (Supersonic). For each method usable in NAFLD cases, we will review the method principle, examination technique and performance in NAFLD evaluation.

Keywords: nonalcoholic fatty liver disease, fibrosis, steatosis, noninvasive, elastography

1. Introduction

An increasingly common cause of chronic liver disease in adults and children is nonalcoholic fatty liver disease (NAFLD) [1]. In adults, the prevalence of NAFLD ranges from 17% to 33% [2], whereas in children, from 2.6% to 9.6%; in obese children, the prevalence is significantly higher: 22.5%–44% [3]. NAFLD may present in various ways: as simple steatosis, nonalcoholic steatohepatitis, liver cirrhosis or even hepatocellular carcinoma (HCC) [2–5].

The diagnosis of NAFLD was traditionally based on the histopathological changes of the liver, evaluated by needle liver biopsy (LB). Unfortunately, this is an invasive method, with potential adverse effects and great inter and intraobserver variability [6–8]. In addition, the interpretation may be erroneous, because of the inhomogeneous distribution of fibrosis. In patients with HCV infection, for instance, differences of at least 1 stage between the right and left lobe in 33% of cases [7] or between 2 samples taken from the same area in even up to 45% of cases have been reported in literature [9]. In patients with nonalcoholic steatohepatitis (NASH), the inhomogeneous distribution of fibrosis appears to be even more pronounced than in HCV patients [10]. Some studies [8] showed that, when taking 2 samples from the right hepatic lobe in each NASH patient, agreement in fibrosis stage was found in only 47% of patients, while differences of at least 1 stage were found in 41% of cases, or 2 stages, in 12% of cases, respectively.

Lately, patients with NASH are increasingly evaluated using rapid, noninvasive methods of assessment of both fibrosis and steatosis. The diagnosis of liver steatosis has several implications in chronic liver diseases [11]. Indeed, in HCV patients, for instance, liver steatosis is associated with fibrosis progression and a decreased rate of sustained viral response [11–13]. Steatosis (which is the primary lesion in nonalcoholic fatty liver disease) may associate graft failure 1 year after liver transplantation, with increased risk of complications after liver resection and, last but not least, increased risk of death [11, 14–16].

The fibrosis may be assessed noninvasively using serum biomarkers (not liver-specific, but proven to correlate with fibrosis), as well as by measuring certain intrinsic physical properties of the liver parenchyma, such as liver stiffness (LS) or shear wave velocity (SWV) within the liver [17]. Of these noninvasive methods, in this chapter, we will focus on the methods assessing the stiffness of liver parenchyma, i.e. elastographic methods, of which, the most widely used are ultrasound (US) elastography techniques.

2. Classification of US-based elastography techniques

Elastography may be considered "a type of remote palpation that allows measurement and display of biomechanical properties associated with the elastic restoring forces in the tissue that act against shear deformation" [18].

In accordance to the European Federation of Societies for Ultrasound in Medicine and Biology (EFSUMB) Guidelines [19, 20], the ultrasound elastographic techniques are either quantitative (shear wave elastography, SWE) or qualitative (strain elastography, real-time elastography). The quantitative techniques are as follows:

- Transient elastography (TE), the only method nonintegrated into a standard ultrasound system.
- Point SWE: Acoustic radiation force impulse elastography (ARFI) or ElastPQ technique.
- Real time SWE: Two-dimensional SWE (2D-SWE) or three-dimensional SWE (3D-SWE)

In the following sections, we will focus on the main quantitative ultrasound elastography techniques, which can help in the noninvasive assessment of nonalcoholic fatty liver disease.

3. Transient elastography (TE)

3.1. Principle

Transient elastography is performed using the Fibroscan® device (Echosens, Paris). The transducer of the device is placed in an intercostal space, above the right lobe, in a point of maximal hepatic dullness (typically the 9–11th intercostal space, on the midaxillary line). A mechanical vibrator is mounted on the axis of the transducer; the vibrator generates a painless vibration, inducing a train of elastic waves, which propagate through the skin and subcutaneous tissue to the liver. In parallel to the vibration, the transducer performs ultrasound acquisitions, at a frequency of 4 kHz. By comparing the ultrasonographic signals thus obtained, tissue deformation records, induced by the propagation of the elastic wave, can be drawn. The time necessary for the train of waves to propagate along the interest area, as well as the velocity of propagation, is recorded [21–25]. The liver stiffness may therefore be calculated using the formula: $E = 3\rho Vs^2$ (E—elasticity modulus; ρ—density, a constant of the material; Vs—the elastic wave propagation velocity within the liver parenchyma). Young's modulus (E) clinically corresponds to the LS and is typically referred to as E or LS. LS values range from 2.5 to 75 kPa. The stiffer the tissue, the higher the train wave propagation velocity [1, 24]. Lower values indicate a more elastic liver.

On the other hand, knowing that fat affects ultrasound propagation, a novel attenuation parameter has been developed to detect and quantify liver steatosis [25]. This parameter, called controlled attenuation parameter (CAP), is based on the ultrasonic properties of the radiofrequency back propagated signals acquired by the Fibroscan® [26]. This ultrasonic attenuation coefficient is an estimate of the total ultrasonic attenuation (go-and-return path) at the central frequency of the regular or M probe of the Fibroscan® probe, i.e. at 3.5 MHz, and is expressed in dB/m and ranges from 100 to 400 dB/m. CAP is evaluated using the same radiofrequency data, and the same region of interest, as the region used to assess the LS [26, 27]. It follows that the equipment can measure the liver stiffness (for the estimation of fibrosis) at the same time with CAP (for the estimation of steatosis) [25].

3.2. Examination technique

The patient is placed in a dorsal decubitus position, with the right arm in maximum abduction, in order to best expose the right quadrant, and the transducer is placed in direct contact with the skin, perpendicularly to the intercostal space, in an area of maximal dullness, free of any large vascular structure. The correct position is ensured either by visualizing the image of the A mode of the system or by using a different ultrasound equipment [22, 24].

When pressing the transducer button, the vibration is generated and transmitted to the liver. The software of the equipment analyses the tissue deformation records and measures the stiffness of the parenchyma. The results are expressed in kiloPascals (kPa) and represent the median value of 10 valid measurements [22, 24]. At the same time, the software can measure the controlled attenuation parameter (CAP), expressed in dB/m.

The monitor of the device will display the instantaneous liver stiffness and CAP values, the median stiffness and CAP values resulting for each of the 10 valid measurements, the measurement success rate as well as the variation of the 10 measurements from the median (IQR).

A necessary condition for a correct assessment is the examination after an overnight fast or at least 2 hours after a meal, because a postprandial examination would increase the stiffness value due to increased hepatic blood flow [28, 29] and would lead to a false interpretation of liver stiffness. The influence of postprandial examination on CAP has not yet been proven.

The measurement can be performed even by a technician after a training period (approximately 100 cases) [30, 31], but the clinical interpretation of results must always be issued by an expert taking into account the demographic data, disease etiology and biochemical profile at the moment of the examination [32].

3.3. Parameters of the examination performance

In accordance to the manufacturer recommendations, the success rate is required to reach at least 60%, and the IQR to be less than 30% of the median (M) liver stiffness [24], although it appears that the best concordance with the biopsy is obtained when its value does not exceed 20% of the median [33].

According to the latest reports, however, the conventional definition of LS measurement accuracy is not relevant. The "success rate ≥ 60%" parameter is considered to be no longer necessary, and the examination accuracy depends on the IQR/M ratio, influenced by the median LS value. Three categories of measurement performance are therefore defined [34]:

- "very reliable": IQR/M ≤ 0.10
- "reliable": 0.10 < IQR/M ≤ 0.30 or IQR/M > 0.30 and LS <7.1 kPa
- "poorly reliable": IQR/M > 0.30 and LS ≥ 7.1 kPa

3.4. The liver volume examined by TE

The technique can measure the stiffness of a cylinder of parenchyma with a 1 cm diameter and a 4 cm height (the measurement is performed on a distance ranging from 25 and 45 mm from the skin); this represents around 1/500 of the entire liver volume, which is at least 100 times larger than the volume of a biopsy sample [22, 30, 32].

3.5. TE reproducibility

TE has a high degree of reproducibility, with a 0.93–0.98 intraobserver and interobserver correlation coefficient [35, 36]. Interobserver concordance is lower in patients with early stages of fibrosis, in those with ≥25% steatosis and in patients with BMI ≥25 kg/m^2.

http://dx.doi.org/10.5772/intechopen.71161

3.6. Normal range of liver stiffness

The mean value of liver stiffness in healthy subjects without any known liver disease and with normal biochemistry and hematology tests is 5.5 ± 1.6 kPa according to some authors [37] and 4.8 ± 1.3 kPa according to others [38]. Age does not appear to influence this value, but stiffness is higher in men than in women. It is very difficult to establish the normal range of liver stiffness without biopsy, but the reverse is not feasible. In a group of HCV patients, without pathological changes on the biopsy sample, the liver stiffness was 4.84 ± 1.49 kPa [39]. In our unit, values of or above 5.3 kPa have a positive predictive value of 90% for the prediction of a fibrosis stage of at least F1.

3.7. Pathological changes influencing liver stiffness in NASH

Our studies performed on a group of biopsied NASH patients proved that LS correlated moderately with fibrosis ($r = 0.661$; $p < 0.0001$) and weakly, but significantly, with hepatocyte ballooning ($r = 0.385$; $p = 0.001$), lobular inflammation ($r = 0.364$; $p = 0.002$) and steatosis ($r = 0.435$; $p < 0.0001$). Of all of these elements, fibrosis was found in a multivariate analysis to be the only factor independently influencing LS in NASH patients [40]. Nevertheless, the correlation between liver stiffness and fibrosis is weaker in NASH ($r = 0.661$) than in hepatitis C ($r = 0.73$–0.79) [41, 42]; this correlation is supported also by the computerized analysis of the biopsy sample that quantifies the amount of fibrosis on the entire sample [43] and is explained by a different distribution pattern of fibrosis in the two conditions [40, 43].

3.8. Diagnostic performance of TE in quantifying fibrosis and steatosis in NASH

Unlike studies performed on diffuse liver diseases of viral etiology, those assessing the role of TE in evaluating NASH patients are rather scarce.

Although liver stiffness is strongly correlated with fibrosis in chronic hepatitis patients, this correlation is weaker in patients with steatohepatitis, because of a different pattern of fibrosis distribution, which, as mentioned earlier, leads to a lower performance of this technique in fibrosis prediction in NASH. Indeed, we observed that liver stiffness in NASH increases alongside the fibrosis stage, but there appears to be an apparent overlap of LS values, especially for the F1-F2 patients [40].

In a meta-analysis including 854 NASH patients [44], TE was found to have a very good performance in diagnosing stages $F \geq 3$ (Se 82%, Sp 82%) and F4 (Se 92%, Sp 92%), but only moderate in diagnosing significant fibrosis $F \geq 2$ (Se 79%, Sp 75%).

The cut-off values for the prediction of fibrosis resulting from various studies differ considerably in NAFLD patients, due to the different prevalence of fibrosis stages in the analyzed groups, as well as to the aim of the analysis (sensibility >90% or specificity >90% or a maximal diagnostic accuracy). Therefore, the proposed cut-offs range between 5.3 and 7 kPa (for $F \geq 1$), with 61.7–93.48% sensitivity and 68–100% specificity (**Table 1**); 5.8–11 kPa (for $F \geq 2$), with 52.5–91.1% sensitivity and 50.3–91.7% specificity (**Table 2**); 7.8–12 kPa (for $F \geq 3$), with 75–100% sensitivity and 78–96.87% specificity (**Table 3**) and between 10.2 and 20 kPa

≥F1	Cut-off (kPa)	AUROC	Se (%)	Sp (%)	PPV (%)	NPV (%)
Yoneda et al. [45]	5.9	0,93	86.1	88.9	97.1	59.3
Lupsor et al. [40]	5.3	0.879	93.48	78.26	89.6	85.7
Kumar et al. [46]	6.1	0.82	78	68	87	53
Imajo et al. [47]	7	0.78	61.7	100	100	86.6

Table 1. Performance of liver stiffness measurement compared with liver biopsy in the detection of fibrosis ≥F1 in nonalcoholic fatty liver disease patients.

(for the prediction of cirrhosis), with 70–100% sensitivity and 68–96.6% specificity (**Table 4**) [40, 45–50]. The studies have shown that TE performance is better for cirrhosis than for significant fibrosis [51, 52].

The available data indicate that, in patients with NAFLD, TE is a highly accurate, noninvasive method for the exclusion of advanced fibrosis and a moderately accurate method for the exclusion of significant fibrosis. According to the EFSUMB and EASL Guidelines and Recommendations on the Clinical Use of Liver Ultrasound Elastography, TE can be used in NAFLD patients to confidently exclude severe fibrosis and especially cirrhosis, with a high negative predictive value (around 90%) [17, 18].

The major challenge for the use of transient elastography in patients with NAFLD in clinical practice is the high rate of failure (no valid shot) or unreliable results (not meeting the manufacturer's first recommendations). In these patients, the failure rate varies between 3.8 and 50% [40, 45, 48, 51, 53–56] and appears to be correlated mainly with obesity [57]. In fact, different studies report increased failure rates owing to increased body mass index (BMI > 30 kg/m^2) or waist circumference, which may interfere with the transmission of the push impulses and the tracking ultrasound, thus preventing a correct estimation of liver stiffness [17]. Apart from

≥F2	Cut-off (kPa)	AUROC	Se (%)	Sp (%)	PPV (%)	NPV (%)
Yoneda et al. [45]	6.65	0.865	88.2	73.9	78.9	85
Lupsor et al. [40]	6.8	0.789	66.67	84.31	60	87.8
Wong et al. [48]	5.8 (Sn > 90%)	0.84	91.1	50.3	56.1	89.0
	7 (max DA)		79.2	75.9	69.6	84.0
	9 (Sp > 90%)		52.5	91.7	81.5	73.5
Kumar et al. [46]	7	0.85	77	78	75	81
Pathik et al. [49]	9.1	—	—	—	—	—
Imajo et al. [47]	11	0.82	65.2	88.7	88.2	66.2
Cassinotto et al. [50]	8.5	0.82	72	79	—	—

Table 2. Performance of liver stiffness measurement compared with liver biopsy in the detection of fibrosis ≥F2 in nonalcoholic fatty liver disease patients.

≥F3	Cut-off (kPa)	AUROC	Se (%)	Sp (%)	PPV (%)	NPV (%)
Yoneda et al. [45]	9.8	0.904	85.2	81.4	63.9	93
Lupsor et al. [40]	10.2	0.978	100	96.87	71.4	100
Wong et al. [48]	7.9 (Sn > 90%)	0.93	91.1	75.3	52.0	96.6
	8.7 (max DA)		83.9	83.2	59.5	94.6
	9.6 (Sp > 90%)		75.0	91.6	72.4	92.6
Kumar et al. [46]	9 (Se + Sp max)	0.94	85	88	68	95
	7.8 (Sn > 90%)		96	78	43	98
	11.2 (Sp > 90%)		71	93	57	91
Pathik et al. [49]	12	—	90	80	—	—
Cassinotto et al. [50]	9.3	0.86	82	75	NR	NR
Imajo et al. [47]	11.4	0.88	85.7	83.8	75	91.9

Table 3. Performance of liver stiffness measurement compared with liver biopsy in the detection of fibrosis ≥F3 in nonalcoholic fatty liver disease patients.

obesity, measurement failure correlates also with more general features of the metabolic syndrome, as well as with limited operator experience [57].

A new transient elastography probe (XL) has been proposed to overcome these limitations for patients who are overweight or obese [54, 55, 58–60]. While the M probe, with a transducer central frequency of 3.5 MHz, can be used when the skin-to-liver capsule distance <2.5 cm (measurement depth 2.5–6.5 cm), the XL probe has a transducer central frequency of 2.5 MHz, so that the LS measurement can be made at a depth of 3.5–7.5 cm and, therefore, can be used

F4	Cut-off (kPa)	AUROC	Se (%)	Sp (%)	PPV (%)	NPV (%)
Yoneda et al. [45]	17.5	0.991	100	96.6	75	100
Wong et al. [48]	10.3 (Sn > 90%)	0.95	92.0	87.8	46.0	99.0
	10.3 (max DA)		92.0	87.8	46.0	99.0
	11.5 (Sp > 90%)		76.0	91.0	48.7	97.1
Kumar et al. [46]	11.8 (Se + Sp max)	0.96	90	88	41	98
	10.6 (Sn > 90%)		100	82	33	100
	19.4 (Sp > 90%)		70	98	78	97
Pathik et al. [49]	20	NR	90	80	NR	NR
Imajo et al. [47]	14	0.92	100	75.9	73	100
Cassinotto et al. [50]	10.2	0.87	89	68	NR	NR

Table 4. Performance of liver stiffness measurement compared with liver biopsy in the detection of cirrhosis in nonalcoholic fatty liver disease patients.

when the skin-to-liver capsule distance ranges between 2.5 and 3.5 cm. The measurement failure is significantly less frequent when using the XL probe than the standard M probe (1.1% versus 16%; $p < 0.00005$) [54]. Unreliable results were still observed with the XL probe, but only in 25%, as opposed to 50% of cases with the M probe ($p < 0.00005$) [57]. The main limiting factors for the XL probe are a skin-to-liver capsule distance >3.4 cm and extreme obesity (BMI > 40 kg/m^2) [54].

It is worth mentioning that, when measured with the XL probe, the median LS is significantly lower than that measured with the M probe (6.9 kPa vs. 8.4 kPa, respectively) [55, 58]. In accordance to the existing literature, the LS cut-off values should be approximately 1.5–2 kPa lower for the same stage of fibrosis when the XL probe is used rather than the M probe [1]. As a result, the cut-off values defined for the M probe cannot be applied to the XL probe, as well.

3.9. Follow-up of patients

Monitoring the progression of fibrosis is also necessary in the follow-up of these patients. European Association for Study of Liver and Asociacion Latinoamericana para el Estudio del Higado [17] and some authors [61] have shown that, indeed, LS measurement may be used to monitor hepatic fibrosis severity in patients with NAFLD, but additional prospective studies are necessary [1]. According to the existing guidelines, follow-up assessment by either serum biomarkers or TE for the progression of liver fibrosis should be performed among NAFLD patients at 3-year interval [17].

3.10. Errors of interpretation of LS values

The liver is an organ wrapped in a distensible but nonelastic envelope (Glisson's capsula). As a result, additional tissue abnormalities (edema, inflammation, cholestasis, congestion), may interfere with LS measurements, independently of fibrosis: increased cytolysis [62–64], extrahepatic cholestasis [65], congestive heart failure [66] and food intake [28, 29]. These error factors should be taken into consideration whenever interpreting LS values since they may overestimate the fibrosis stage [57]. The influence of steatosis on liver stiffness is still rather controversial; some studies indicate that steatosis may lead to higher liver stiffness, independently of fibrosis [53, 67], whereas others did not find the same effect [48]. It follows that more studies are needed to clarify this aspect, especially in NAFLD patients examined with both the M and the XL probe.

3.11. Prediction of steatosis in NAFLD patients using CAP measurements

The new parameter, which can be measured using the Fibroscan® equipment, the controlled attenuation parameter (CAP), has proven, in our and other authors' experience, to correlate significantly only with steatosis, not with other pathological anomalies encountered in patients with diffuse liver diseases (inflammation, ballooning or fibrosis) [26, 47, 54, 68–75].

An increase of the CAP value can be seen alongside the increase in steatosis grade, but there is some degree of overlap between adjacent grades, especially between moderate and severe steatosis [68].

The studies on the assessment of CAP performance in grading steatosis were predominantly aimed at groups of patients with various diffuse liver diseases, not only NAFLD. For the prediction of steatosis >10%, the CAP cut-off values vary in different studies between 214 dB/m and 289 dB/m, with a 64–91% sensitivity range and a 64–94% specificity range and the AUROC between 0.68 and 0.91. For the prediction of steatosis >33%, the cut-offs range between 259 dB/m and 311 dB/m, with a 57–89% sensitivity range and a 62–94% specificity range and the AUROC between 0.73 and 0.95. For the prediction of severe steatosis (>66%), the cut-offs range between 281 dB/m and 318 dB/m, with a 71–100% sensitivity range and a 47–82.5% specificity range and the AUROC between 0.70 and 0.93 [26, 47, 68–76]. According to these studies, CAP is useful in the detection of $S \geq 10\%$, $S \geq 33\%$ and $S \geq 66\%$, as a result of its good sensitivity and specificity; however, the exact cut-off values remain to be defined [1].

A recent meta-analysis including 2735 patients, 20% having NAFLD [77], has established the optimal CAP cut-offs for the prediction of mild, moderate and severe steatosis as, respectively, 248 dB/m, 268 dB/m, and 280 dB/m, with 66.8%, 77.3%, respectively 88.2% sensibility, and 82.2%, 81.2%, respectively 77.6% specificity (**Table 5**). According to this meta-analysis [77], covariates such as etiology, BMI and diabetes should be taken into account when interpreting CAP, but sex, age and fibrosis play a much smaller role. The authors recommend using the cut-offs established here, but deducting 10 dB/m from the CAP value for NAFLD/NASH patients, 10 dB/m for diabetes patients and deducting or adding 4.4 dB/m for each unit of BMI above or below 25 kg/m^2 over the range of 20–30 kg/m^2 [77].

In conclusion, CAP is a noninvasive method for the assessment of steatosis in chronic liver disease patients, including NASH, with a diagnosis accuracy of 76.11–82.06% [68], which is independently influenced only by the amount of steatosis. Due to its negative predictive value of 93.5–98.7%, CAP could become a useful clinical tool especially in excluding significant steatosis grades [68]. Large studies are required in order to develop new cut-off values for liver

	S0 vs. S1–S3	**S0–S1 vs. S2–S3**	**S0–S2 vs. S3**
Optimal cut off, dB/m	248 (237–261)	268 (257–284)	280 (268–294)
AUC	0.823 (0.809–0.837)	0.865 (0.850–0.880)	0.882 (0.858–0.906)
Sensitivity	0.688 (0.600–0.750)	0.773 (0.690–0.838)	0.882 (0.765–0.956)
False negative rate	0.312 (0.250–0.400)	0.227 (0.162–0.310)	0.118 (0.044–0.235)
Specificity	0.822 (0.761–0.897)	0.812 (0.749–0.879)	0.776 (0.720–0.821)
False positive rate	0.178 (0.103–0.239)	0.188 (0.121–0.251)	0.224 (0.179–0.280)

Table 5. Optimal CAP cut-off values, based on the maximal sum of sensitivity and specificity (Youden index) in predicting steatosis (modified after Karlas et al. [77]).

fibrosis staging using the XL probe and to investigate the differences between the CAP cut-off values used for the M and XL probes [1].

3.12. Advantages of transient elastography with controlled attenuation parameter

TE, the most widely used and validated noninvasive technique, offers several advantages [1, 26, 57, 68, 71]: it is user-friendly, machine-independent and painless, has a short duration of examination and does not require corrections to be made for gain, frequency, focusing or beam diffraction. This technique is highly reproducible, has well-defined quality criteria and allows the simultaneous assessment of liver stiffness (for fibrosis) and CAP (for steatosis) in the same region of the liver. Compared to liver biopsy, the technique is less prone to sampling errors as it explores a liver volume about 100 times larger. Furthermore, the method also has several clinical applications for patients with NAFLD.

3.13. Limitations of transient elastography with controlled attenuation parameter

TE does have some limitations [1], which may lead to measurement failure: ascites (the vibrations do not propagate through liquids), obesity (especially at BMI > 30 kg/m^2) and narrow intercostal spaces. On the other hand, however, some of these limitations may be overcome by using the XL probe (for obese patients) and the S probe (for children). Another limitation of the technique is the overestimation of fibrosis because of increased liver stiffness due to high cytolysis, extrahepatic cholestasis and congestive heart failure.

3.14. Conclusion about the use of TE in NAFLD

In conclusion, TE may prove useful to NAFLD patients especially for the exclusion of significant fibrosis and cirrhosis. However, we must consider the rather high rate of measurement failure in these patients. The XL probe may overcome this problem in obese patients, but new cut-offs should be defined for the prediction of fibrosis, since the ones of the M probe are not applicable for the XL one [1, 57]. Follow-up assessment by TE for the progression of liver fibrosis should be performed among NAFLD patients at 3-year interval [17].

On the other hand, CAP provides a standardized noninvasive measure of hepatic steatosis. According to the latest and most comprehensive meta-analysis [77], the optimal cut-offs for the prediction of mild, moderate and severe steatosis are 248, 268, and 280 dB/m, respectively. Some authors recommend using the cut-offs established here, but deducting 10 dB/m from the CAP value for NAFLD/NASH patients, 10 dB/m for diabetes patients and deducting or adding 4.4 dB/m for each unit of BMI above or below 25 kg/m^2 over the range of 20–30 kg/m^2 [77]. Longitudinal data are needed to demonstrate how CAP relates to clinical outcomes.

4. Acoustic radiation force impulse elastography (ARFI)

Of the "Point SWE" techniques, we will review some features of the ARFI technique (acoustic radiation force impulse elastography), the only technique in this category whose role in the assessment of NAFLD patients has, albeit insufficiently, been analyzed.

4.1. Principle

The ARFI imaging technology involves the mechanical excitation of tissue using short-duration acoustic pulses (push pulses) in a region of interest chosen by the examiner, producing shear waves that spread away from the region of interest, perpendicularly to the acoustic push pulse, generating localized, micron-scale displacements in the tissue [78–80]. Simultaneously, detection waves of lower intensity than that of the push pulse are generated. The shear wave velocity—SWV (m/s) can be calculated taking into account the place and moment of interaction between the shear waves and the detection waves [80–83]. The stiffer the tissue, the higher the shear wave velocity [80–83]. The shear wave velocity is measured in a smaller volume than in transient elastography (10 mm long and 6 mm wide), but, unlike TE, it can be chosen by the operator under B-mode visualization [57], since ARFI is implemented on some ultrasound equipments, alongside the B-mode, color Doppler and contrast modes [17, 80, 84].

4.2. Examination technique

The patient is placed in a dorsal decubitus position, with the right arm in maximum abduction. The transducer is placed in an intercostal space, and the region of interest (10/5 mm) is chosen in an area of the right liver parenchyma (segments 5 or 8), 1–2 cm below the liver capsule; the measurement is performed after asking the patient to hold his/her breath after an expiration to prevent breathing movements [85]. In general, the median value of 10 valid measurements of the shear wave is taken into consideration; sometimes, no valid measurement can be obtained. When taking into account the manufacturer recommendations, we can identify some possible causes, which, alone or in combination, may lead to this situation:

- excessive movements of the liver tissue—for instance, cardiac pulsations transmitted to the liver parenchyma (impaired estimation of shear wave velocity);
- marked signal attenuation in obese patients (impaired identification of the shear wave by the system);
- marked tissue stiffness (impaired estimation of shear wave velocity—shear wave outside of the confidence interval).

On the whole, however, the failure rate of ARFI is significantly lower than that of TE (2.9% vs. 6.4%, $p < 0.001$), especially in patients with ascites or obesity [86].

Ten valid measurements are performed in the right liver lobe, a median value is calculated and the result is expressed in meters/second.

pSWE measurements using Virtual Touch Quantification (VTQ®) in healthy populations range between 1.01 and 1.59 m/s, but in most studies the range is 1.07–1.16 m/s [87–89].

4.3. Errors of interpretation of LS values using the ARFI technique

Like TE, ARFI results are influenced by food intake [90] as well as necroinflammatory activity and aminotransferase levels [91], all of which lead to an overestimation of liver fibrosis and have to be taken into account when interpreting the results [17].

LS values obtained with ARFI, in contrast to TE values, have a narrow range (0.5–4.4 m/s). Defining cut-off values for discriminating certain fibrosis stages is therefore restricted, as well as making management decisions.

4.4. Diagnostic performance of ARFI in NASH

There are few studies assessing the performance of ARFI in NAFLD. The majority of studies included patients with diffuse liver diseases, with only a fraction of NAFLD patients. In most studies, the cut-offs for the prediction of F1 vary between 1.105–1.34 m/s, with 76.7% sensibility and 71.4% specificity; for $F \geq 2$, between 1.137–1.179 m/s, with Se 71–97% and Sp 67–92%; for $F \geq 3$, between 1.45–2.20 m/s, with Se 75–100% and Sp 68–95.2%, and for the prediction of cirrhosis, between 1.61–2.90 m/s, with Se 74–100% and Sp 67–96% [92–98].

ARFI performs better in severe fibrosis and cirrhosis than in significant fibrosis, with AUROCs ranging from 0.91 to 0.98 and from 0.66 to 0.86, respectively [97].

A systematic review of seven studies with a total of 723 patients who underwent shear wave velocity measurements with VTQ® technique to evaluate the diagnostic efficacy of pSWE in patients with NAFLD showed that the summary Se and Sp of ARFI in detecting significant fibrosis were 80.2 and 85.2% [99], which is not an appropriate endpoint [17].

In conclusion, ARFI elastography appears to be modestly accurate in detecting significant fibrosis, but performs well in predicting severe fibrosis and cirrhosis in NAFLD patients. As for its use in the follow-up of patients, no data are available for this technique for the moment.

5. Two-dimensional SWE (2D-SWE)

5.1. Principle

2D-SWE is based on the combination of a radiation force induced in tissues by focused ultrasonic beams and a very high frame rate ultrasound imaging sequence capable of catching in real time the transient propagation of resulting shear waves [17, 19, 100]. The shear wave speed is estimated by a Doppler-like acquisition over a region of interest (ROI) and it is used to calculate the tissue stiffness. The relationship between Young's modulus (E) and the shear wave (c) is $E = 3\rho c^2$ (ρ = tissue density) [19, 20, 100, 101].

The elasticity is displayed using a color-coded image superimposed on a B-mode image: stiffer tissues in red and softer tissues in blue [19, 20, 100, 101]. In addition, a quantitative measurement of the liver stiffness in the chosen region of interest is performed. The equipment allows the visualization of results both in kPa and in m/s, with a maximum value reaching 300 kPa (10 m/s) [102, 103].

Almost all 2D-SWE studies for liver applications have been carried out using Supersonic Imagine equipments (Aixplorer, Supersonic Imagine, Aix en Provence, France), because other companies have only recently introduced 2D-SWE products [17].

5.2. The examination technique

The examination is performed after an overnight fast, with the patient placed in a dorsal decubitus position, with the right arm in maximum abduction, in order to enlarge the intercostal spaces and ensure the best access to the right liver lobe parenchyma [103]. The region of interest (ROI) for the elastography examination is placed in the center of the screen, choosing an homogeneous area of parenchyma, free of any large vascular structure and at least 2 cm below the liver capsule, to prevent any risk of overestimation of fibrosis due to the higher capsular and subcapsular fibrosis content. The ROI with color-coded elastographic information is displayed overlapped on the 2D image; its size can be adjusted up to 3×3 cm, and the depth, although adjustable, should be kept within 8 cm [102].

There is no consensus on the ***number of measurements*** required for a good quality assessment [20]: some studies recommend 3 [104–106], 4 [107] or 5 [108–110].

Similar to pSWE/ARFI, ***quality criteria*** for 2D-SWE remain to be defined. Until now, such criteria have only been proposed in a study on patients with portal hypertension, but they still require validation on prospective studies on large groups of biopsied patients [106]: "highly reliable" (when the ratio between standard deviation/median LS ≤0.10 and measurement depth < 5.6 cm); "reliable" (when standard deviation/median LS >0.10 or measurement depth ≥ 5.6 cm); respectively "unreliable" (when standard deviation/median LS >0.10 and measurement depth ≥ 5.6 cm). The "highly reliable" and "reliable" measurements are considered acceptable; only the "unreliable" ones are considered unacceptable for evaluation and should be rejected [106].

5.3. Technique failure

The liver stiffness cannot be assessed by 2D-SWE in around 10.4% of cases, more frequently in obese patients or in patients with a thoracic wall thicker than 25 mm in the intercostal spaces [111]. Generally speaking, the following factors may be associated with a higher rate of invalid measurements: narrow intercostal spaces [107], high BMI and thoracic wall thicker than 25 mm in the intercostal spaces [111].

5.4. Normal range of liver stiffness as evaluated by 2D-SWE

Studies performed on subjects with healthy livers, pathologically confirmed potential donors, yielded a mean normal value of liver stiffness in 2D-SWE of 4.4–4.9 kPa (range 2.2–6.2 kPa), not correlated significantly with age, BMI or steatosis [100, 105, 107, 109].

5.5. Performance of 2D-SWE in assessing nonalcoholic steatohepatitis

Some studies on the performance of this method in diffuse liver diseases of various etiologies included a certain proportion of NASH patients. The resulting cut-offs varied between 6.2–7.8 kPa for ≥F1, 7.1–10.49 kPa for ≥F2, 8.7–11.5 kPa for ≥F3 and 9.59–18.1 kPa for F4 [112]. 2D-SWE performance for the prediction of each fibrosis stage seems to be similar when including all patients, regardless of etiology, as well as when including only viral hepatic diseases, with AUROCs between 0.80 and 0.82 [103]. In two meta-analyses, with a total of 2303 and 934 patients, respectively, the summary area under the curve (AUC) was 0.85 for ≥F1, 0.87–0.88 for ≥F2, 0.93–0.94 for ≥F3 and 0.92–0.94 for F4 [112, 113].

In a study performed on 291 NAFLD patients, the chosen cut-offs for the prediction of ≥F2 were 6.3 kPa (Se 90%, Sp 50%) and 8.7 kPa (Se 71%, Sp 90%), with AUROC 0.86; for the prediction of fibrosis ≥F3, 8.3 kPa (Se 91%, Sp 71%) and 10.7 kPa (Se 71%, Sp 90%), with AUROC 0.89 and for the prediction of cirrhosis, 10.5 kPa (Se 90%, Sp 72%) and 14.4 kPa (Se 58%, Sp 90%), with AUROC 0.88 [50].

6. Conclusions: SSI, Fibroscan® or ARFI?

After comparing the performance in the assessment of NAFLD of the three elastographic methods discussed above, we can conclude, on the preliminary results, that the diagnostic performance according to the AUROC values for the diagnosis of significant fibrosis, severe fibrosis and cirrhosis is good for SSI (0.86–0.89); good for Fibroscan® (0.82–0.87) and fair or good for ARFI (0.77–0.84) [50]. The AUROC values for diagnosing severe fibrosis or cirrhosis are particularly good for SSI or Fibroscan® (0.86 and 0.89) [50].

The prediction of steatosis, however, can at this moment only be made using the controlled attenuation parameter measured with Fibroscan®.

As for the causes of measurement failure or unreliable results, we mention clinical factors related to obesity (BMI > 30 kg/m^2, waist circumference ≥ 102 cm or increased wall thickness), which are associated with liver stiffness measurement failures when using SSI or Fibroscan® and with unreliable results when using ARFI [50].

In conclusion, SSI, Fibroscan® and ARFI are valuable diagnostic tools for the staging of liver fibrosis in NAFLD patients. However, the diagnostic accuracy of SSI appears to be superior to that of ARFI for the diagnosis of F2 or above [50]. Most of the cut-off values for SSI for the diagnosis of different stages of liver disease are quite similar to those of Fibroscan®; this is an issue of great importance for the applicability of this technique and its wide dissemination among radiologists and hepatologists in their daily practice. However, as for the M probe of Fibroscan®, the SSI technique remains limited by a high failure rate in cases of obesity, whereas ARFI has a high rate of unreliable results [50].

Acknowledgements

This work was supported by a grant of the Romanian National Authority for Scientific Research and Innovation, CNCS – UEFISCDI, project number PN-II-RU-TE-2014-4-2023.

Author details

Monica Lupsor-Platon

Address all correspondence to: monica.lupsor@umfcluj.ro

Department of Medical Imaging, Iuliu Hatieganu University of Medicine and Pharmacy, Regional Institute of Gastroenterology and Hepatology "Prof. Dr. Octavian Fodor", Cluj-Napoca, Romania

References

[1] Mikolasevic I, Orlic L, Franjic N, Hauser G, Stimac D, Milic S. Transient elastography (FibroScan(®)) with controlled attenuation parameter in the assessment of liver steatosis and fibrosis in patients with nonalcoholic fatty liver disease—Where do we stand? World Journal of Gastroenterology. 2016;**22**(32):7236-7251. DOI: 10.3748/wjg.v22.i32.7236

[2] Bang KB, Cho YK. Comorbidities and metabolic derangement of NAFLD. Journal of Lifestyle Medicine. 2015;**5**(1):7-13. DOI: 10.15280/jlm.2015.5.1.7

[3] Cho Y, Tokuhara D, Morikawa H, Kuwae Y, Hayashi E, Hirose M, et al. Transient elastography-based liver profiles in a hospital-based pediatric population in Japan. PLoS One. 2015;**10**(9):e0137239. DOI: 10.1371/journal.pone.0137239

[4] Byrne CD, Targher GNAFLD. A multisystem disease. Journal of Hepatology. 2015;**62** (1 Suppl):S47-S64. DOI: 10.1016/j.jhep.2014.12.012

[5] Smits MM, Ioannou GN, Boyko EJ, Utzschneider KM. Non-alcoholic fatty liver disease as an independent manifestation of the metabolic syndrome: Results of a US national survey in three ethnic groups. Journal of Gastroenterology and Hepatology. 2013;**28**(4):664-670. DOI: 10.1111/jgh.12106

[6] Bedossa P, Dargère D, Paradis V. Sampling variability of liver fibrosis in chronic hepatitis C. Hepatology. 2003;**38**(6):1449-1457. DOI: 10.1016/j.hep.2003.09.022

[7] Regev A, Berho M, Jeffers LJ, Milikowski C, Molina EG, Pyrsopoulos NT, et al. Sampling error and intraobserver variation in liver biopsy in patients with chronic HCV infection. The American Journal of Gastroenterology. 2002;**97**(10):2614-2618. DOI: 10.1111/j.1572-0241.2002.06038.x

[8] Ratziu V, Charlotte F, Heurtier A, Gombert S, Giral P, Bruckert E, et al. Sampling variability of liver biopsy in nonalcoholic fatty liver disease. Gastroenterology. 2005;**128**(7):1898-1906. DOI: http://dx.doi.org/10.1053/j.gastro.2005.03.084

[9] Siddique I, El-Naga HA, Madda JP, Memon A, Hasan F. Sampling variability on percutaneous liver biopsy in patients with chronic hepatitis C virus infection. Scandinavian Journal of Gastroenterology. 2003;**38**(4):427-432

[10] Goldstein NS, Hastah F, Galan MV, Gordon SC. Fibrosis heterogeneity in nonalcoholic steatohepatitis and hepatitis C virus needle core biopsy specimens. American Journal of Clinical Pathology. 2005;**123**(3):382-387. DOI: 10.1309/EY72-F1EN-9XCB-1KXX

[11] Boursier J, Calès P. Controlled attenuation parameter (CAP): A new device for fast evaluation of liver fat? Liver International. 2012;**32**(6):875-877. DOI: 10.1111/j.1478-3231.2012.02824.x

[12] Leandro G, Mangia A, Hui J, Fabris P, Rubbia-Brandt L, Colloredo G, et al. HCV Meta-Analysis (on) Individual Patients' Data Study Group. Relationship between steatosis, inflammation, and fibrosis in chronic hepatitis C: A meta-analysis of individual patient data. Gastroenterology. 2006;**130**:1636-1642. DOI: http://dx.doi.org/10.1053/j.gastro.2006.03.014

[13] Poynard T, Ratziu V, McHutchison J, Manns M, Goodman Z, Zeuzem S, et al. Effect of treatment with peginterferon or interferon alfa-2b and ribavirin on steatosis in patients infected with hepatitis C. Hepatology. 2003;**38**(1):75-85. DOI: 10.1053/jhep.2003.50267

[14] Spitzer AL, Lao OB, Dick AA, Bakthavatsalam R, Halldorson JB, Yeh MM, Upton MP, Reyes JD, Perkins JD. The biopsied donor liver: Incorporating macrosteatosis into high-risk donor assessment. Liver Transplantation. 2010;**16**:874-884. DOI: 10.1002/lt.22085

[15] de Meijer VE, Kalish BT, Puder M, Ijzermans JN. Systematic review and meta-analysis of steatosis as a risk factor in major hepatic resection. The British Journal of Surgery. 2010;**97**:1331-1339. DOI: 10.1002/bjs.7194

[16] Younossi ZM, Stepanova M, Afendy M, Fang Y, Younossi Y, Mir H, et al. Changes in the prevalence of the most common causes of chronic liver diseases in the United States from 1988 to 2008. Clinical Gastroenterology and Hepatology. 2011;**9**:524-530. DOI: 10.1016/j.cgh.2011.03.020

[17] European Association for Study of Liver; Asociacion Latinoamericana para el Estudio del Higado. EASL-ALEH clinical practice guidelines: Non-invasive tests for evaluation of liver disease severity and prognosis. Journal of Hepatology. 2015;**63**(1):237-264. DOI: 10.1016/j.jhep.2015.04.006

[18] Dietrich CF, Bamber J, Berzigotti A, Bota S, Cantisani V, Castera L, et al. EFSUMB guidelines and recommendations on the clinical use of liver ultrasound elastography, update 2017 (long version). Ultraschall Med. 2017:**38**(4):e16-e47. DOI: 10.1055/s-0043-103952

[19] Bamber J, Cosgrove D, Dietrich CF, Fromageau J, Bojunga J, Calliada F, et al. EFSUMB guidelines and recommendations on the clinical use of ultrasound elastography. Part 1: Basic principles and technology. Ultraschall in der Medizin. 2013;**34**(2):169-184. DOI: 10.1055/s-0033-1335205

[20] Sporea I, Bota S, Săftoiu A, Şirli R, Gradinăru-Taşcău O, Popescu A, et al. Romanian national guidelines and practical recommendations on liver elastography. Medical Ultrasonography. 2014;**16**(2):123-138. DOI: 10.11152/mu.2013.2066.162.is1sb2

[21] Lupşor M, Badea R. Elastografia unidimensională tranzitorie. In Badea R, Dudea S, Mircea PM. Stamate M. Tratat de Ultrasonografie clinică, Vol III. Bucuresti: Ed Medicala; 2008. pp. 675-685

[22] Lupşor M, Badea R, Stefănescu H. Evaluarea neinvazivă a fibrozei hepatice. In: Pascu O, Grigorescu M, Acalovschi M, Andreica V, editors. Gastroenterologie. Hepatologie – Bazele practicii clinice. Cluj Napoca: Ed. Medicală Universitară Iuliu Haţieganu; 2010. pp. 402-408

[23] Yeh WC, Li PC, Jeng YM, Hsu HC, Kuo PL, Li ML, et al. Elastic modulus measurements of human liver and correlation with pathology. Ultrasound in Medicine & Biology. 2002;**28**(4):467-474

[24] Sandrin L, Fourquet B, Hasquenoph JM, Yon S, Fournier C, Mal F, et al. Transient elastography: A new noninvasive method for assessment of hepatic fibrosis. Ultrasound in Medicine&Biology. 2003;**29**(12):1705-1713. DOI: http://dx.doi.org/10.1016/j.ultrasmedbio.2003.07.001

[25] Lupsor M, Stefanescu H, Feier D, Badea R. Non-invasive evaluation of liver steatosis, fibrosis and cirrhosis in hepatitis C virus infected patients using unidimensional transient elastography (Fibroscan®). In: Tagaya N, editor. Liver Biopsy—Indications, Procedures, Results. Croatia: Intech; 2012. pp. 209-234. DOI: 10.5772/52621

[26] Sasso M, Beaugrand M, de Ledinghen V, Douvin C, Marcellin P, Poupon R, et al. Controlled attenuation parameter (CAP): A novel VCTE™ guided ultrasonic attenuation measurement for the evaluation of hepatic steatosis: Preliminary study and validation in a cohort of patients with chronic liver disease from various causes. Ultrasound in Medicine & Biology. 2010;**36**(11):1825-1835. DOI: 10.1016/j.ultrasmedbio.2010.07.005

[27] Sasso M, Miette V, Sandrin L, Beaugrand M. The controlled attenuation parameter (CAP): A novel tool for the non-invasive evaluation of steatosis using Fibroscan. Clinics and Research in Hepatology and Gastroenterology. 2012;**36**(1):13-20. DOI: 10.1016/j.clinre.2011.08.001

[28] Mederacke I, Wursthorn K, Kirschner J, Rifai K, Manns MP, Wedemeyer H, et al. Food intake increases liver stiffness in patients with chronic or resolved hepatitis C virus infection. Liver International. 2009;**29**(10):1500-1506. DOI: 10.1111/j.1478-3231.2009.02100.x

[29] Arena U, Lupsor Platon M, Stasi C, Moscarella S, Assarat A, Bedogni G, et al. Liver stiffness is influenced by a standardized meal in patients with chronic hcv hepatitis at different stages of fibrotic evolution. Hepatology. 2013;**58**(1):65-72. DOI: 10.1002/hep.26343

[30] Kettaneh A, Marcellin P, Douvin C, Poupon R, Ziol M, Beaugrand M, et al. Features associated with success rate and performance of FibroScan measurements for the diagnosis of cirrhosis in HCV patients: A prospective study of 935 patients. Journal of Hepatology. 2007;**46**(4):628-634. DOI: http://dx.doi.org/10.1016/j.jhep.2006.11.010

[31] Boursier J, Konate A, Guilluy M, Gorea G, Sawadogo A, Quemener E, et al. Learning curve and interobserver reproducibility evaluation of liver stiffness measurement by transient

elastography. European Journal of Gastroenterology & Hepatology. 2008;**20**(7):693-701. DOI: 10.1097/MEG.0b013e3282f51992

[32] Castera L, Forns X, Alberti A. Non-invasive evaluation of liver fibrosis using transient elastography. Journal of Hepatology. 2008;**48**(5):835-847. DOI: 10.1016/j.jhep.2008.02.008

[33] Lucidarme D, Foucher J, Le Bail B, Vergniol J, Castera L, Duburque C, et al. Factors of accuracy of transient elastography (fibroscan) for the diagnosis of liver fibrosis in chronic hepatitis C. Hepatology. 2008;**49**(4):1083-1089. DOI: 10.1002/hep.22748

[34] Boursier J, Zarski JP, de Ledinghen V, Rousselet MC, Sturm N, Lebail B, et al. Determination of reliability criteria for liver stiffness evaluation by transient elastography. Hepatology. 2013;**57**(3):1182-1191. DOI: 10.1002/hep.25993

[35] Fraquelli M, Rigamonti C, Casazza G, Conte D, Donato MF, Ronchi G, et al. Reproducibility of transient elastography in the evaluation of liver fibrosis in patients with chronic liver disease. Gut. 2007;**56**(7):968-973. DOI: 10.1136/gut.2006.111302

[36] Boursier J, Konaté A, Gorea G, Reaud S, Quemener E, Oberti F, et al. Reproducibility of liver stiffness measurement by ultrasonographic elastometry. Clinical Gastroenterology and Hepatology. 2008;**6**(11):1263-1269. DOI: 10.1016/j.cgh.2008.07.006

[37] Roulot D, Czernichow S, Le Clésiau H, Costes JL, Vergnaud AC, Beaugrand M. Liver stiffness values in apparently healthy subjects: Influence of gender and metabolic syndrome. Journal of Hepatology. 2008;**48**(4):606-613. DOI: 10.1016/j.jhep.2007.11.020

[38] Sirli R, Sporea I, Tudora A, Deleanu A, Popescu A. Transient elastographic evaluation of subjects without known hepatic pathology: Does age change the liver stiffness? Journal of Gastrointestinal and Liver Diseases. 2009;**18**(1):57-60

[39] Lupsor Platon M, Stefanescu H, Feier D, Maniu A, Badea R. Performance of unidimensional transient elastography in staging chronic hepatitis C. Results from a cohort of 1,202 biopsied patients from one single center. Journal of Gastrointestinal and Liver Diseases. 2013;**22**(2):157-166

[40] Lupsor M, Badea R, Stefanescu H, Grigorescu M, Serban A, Radu C. Performance of unidimensional transient elastography in staging non-alcoholic steatohepatitis. Journal of Gastrointestinal and Liver Diseases. 2010;**19**(1):53-60

[41] Lupşor M, Badea R, Stefănescu H, Grigorescu M, Sparchez Z, Serban A, et al. Analysis of histopathological changes that influence liver stiffness in chronic hepatitis C. Results from a cohort of 324 patients. Journal of Gastrointestinal and Liver Diseases. 2008;**17**:155-163

[42] Foucher J, Chanteloup E, Vergniol J, Castéra L, Le Bail B, Adhoute X, et al. Diagnosis of cirrhosis by transient elastography (FibroScan): A prospective study. Gut. 2006;**55**:403-408. DOI: 10.1136/gut.2005.069153

[43] Ziol M, Kettaneh A, Ganne-Carrié N, Barget N, Tengher-Barna I, Beaugrand M. Relationships between fibrosis amounts assessed by morphometry and liver stiffness measurements in

chronic hepatitis or steatohepatitis. European Journal of Gastroenterology & Hepatology. 2009;**21**:1261-1268. DOI: 10.1097/MEG.0b013e32832a20f5

[44] Kwok R, Tse YK, Wong GL, Ha Y, Lee AU, Ngu MC, et al. Systematic review with meta-analysis: Non-invasive assessment of non-alcoholic fatty liver disease—The role of transient elastography and plasma cytokeratin-18 fragments. Alimentary Pharmacology & Therapeutics. 2014;**39**(3):254-269. DOI: 10.1111/apt.12569

[45] Yoneda M, Yoneda M, Mawatari H, Fujita K, Endo H, Iida H, et al. Noninvasive assessment of liver fibrosis by measurement of stiffness in patients with nonalcoholic fatty liver disease (NAFLD). Digestive and Liver Disease. 2008;**40**(5):371-378. DOI: http://dx.doi.org/10.1016/j.dld.2007.10.019

[46] Kumar R, Rastogi A, Sharma MK, Bhatia V, Tyagi P, Sharma P, et al. Liver stiffness measurements in patients with different stages of nonalcoholic fatty liver disease: Diagnostic performance and clinicopathological correlation. Digestive Diseases and Sciences. 2013;**58**(1):265-274. DOI: 10.1007/s10620-012-2306-1

[47] Imajo K, Kessoku T, Honda Y, Tomeno W, Ogawa Y, Mawatari H, et al. Magnetic resonance imaging more accurately classifies steatosis and fibrosis in patients with nonalcoholic fatty liver disease than transient elastography. Gastroenterology. 2016;**150**:626-637. DOI: 10.1053/j.gastro.2015.11.048

[48] Wong VW, Vergniol J, Wong GL, Foucher J, Chan HL, Le Bail B, et al. Diagnosis of fibrosis and cirrhosis using liver stiffness measurement in nonalcoholic fatty liver disease. Hepatology. 2010;**51**(2):454-462. DOI: 10.1002/hep.23312

[49] Pathik P, Ravindra S, Ajay C, Prasad B, Jatin P, Prabha S. Fibroscan versus simple noninvasive screening tools in predicting fibrosis in high-risk nonalcoholic fatty liver disease patients from western India. Annals of Gastroenterology. 2015;**28**(2):281-286

[50] Cassinotto C, Boursier J, de Lédinghen V, Lebigot J, Lapuyade B, Cales P, et al. Liver stiffness in nonalcoholic fatty liver disease: A comparison of supersonic shear imaging, FibroScan, and ARFI with liver biopsy. Hepatology. 2016;**63**(6):1817-1827. DOI: 10.1002/hep.28394

[51] Petta S, Vanni E, Bugianesi E, Di Marco V, Cammà C, Cabibi D, et al. The combination of liver stiffness measurement and NAFLD fibrosis score improves the noninvasive diagnostic accuracy for severe liver fibrosis in patients with nonalcoholic fatty liver disease. Liver International. 2015;**35**:1566-1573. DOI: 10.1111/liv.12584

[52] Naveau S, Lamouri K, Pourcher G, Njiké-Nakseu M, Ferretti S, Courie R, et al. The diagnostic accuracy of transient elastography for the diagnosis of liver fibrosis in bariatric surgery candidates with suspected NAFLD. Obesity Surgery. 2014;**24**:1693-1701. DOI: 10.1007/s11695-014-1235-9

[53] Gaia S, Carenzi S, Barilli AL, Bugianesi E, Smedile A, Brunello F, et al. Reliability of transient elastography for the detection of fibrosis in non-alcoholic fatty liver disease

and chronic viral hepatitis. Journal of Hepatology. 2011;**54**(1):64-71. DOI: 10.1016/j.jhep.2010.06.022

[54] Myers RP, Pomier-Layrargues G, Kirsch R, Pollett A, Duarte-Rojo A, Wong D, et al. Feasibility and diagnostic performance of the FibroScan XL probe for liver stiffness measurement in overweight and obese patients. Hepatology. 2012;**55**(1):199-208. DOI: 10.1002/hep.24624

[55] Wong VW, Vergniol J, Wong GL, Foucher J, Chan AW, Chermak F, et al. Liver stiffness measurement using XL probe in patients with nonalcoholic fatty liver disease. The American Journal of Gastroenterology. 2012;**107**(12):1862-1871. DOI: 10.1038/ajg.2012.331

[56] Petta S, Di Marco V, Cammà C, Butera G, Cabibi D, Craxì A. Reliability of liver stiffness measurement in non-alcoholic fatty liver disease: The effects of body mass index. Alimentary Pharmacology & Therapeutics. 2011;**33**(12):1350-1360. DOI: 10.1111/ j.1365-2036.2011.04668.x

[57] Castera L, Vilgrain V, Angulo P. Noninvasive evaluation of NAFLD. Nature Reviews. Gastroenterology & Hepatology. 2013;**10**(11):666-675. DOI: 10.1038/nrgastro.2013

[58] Friedrich-Rust M, Hadji-Hosseini H, Kriener S, Herrmann E, Sircar I, Kau A, et al. Transient elastography with a new probe for obese patients for non-invasive staging of non-alcoholic steatohepatitis. European Radiology. 2010;**20**(10):2390-2396. DOI: 10.1007/s00330-010-1820-9

[59] de Lédinghen V, Vergniol J, Foucher J, El-Hajbi F, Merrouche W, Rigalleau V. Feasibility of liver transient elastography with FibroScan using a new probe for obese patients. Liver International. 2010;**30**(7):1043-1048. DOI: 10.1111/j.1478-3231.2010.02258.x

[60] de Lédinghen V, Wong VW, Vergniol J, Wong GL, Foucher J, Chu SH, et al. Diagnosis of liver fibrosis and cirrhosis using liver stiffness measurement: Comparison between M and XL probe of FibroScan®. Journal of Hepatology. 2012;**56**(4):833-839. DOI: 10.1016/j.jhep.2011.10.017

[61] Suzuki K, Yoneda M, Imajo K, Kirikoshi H, Nakajima A, Maeda S, et al. Transient elastography for monitoring the fibrosis of non-alcoholic fatty liver disease for 4 years. Hepatology Research. 2013;**43**:979-983. DOI: 10.1111/hepr.12039

[62] Coco B, Oliveri F, Maina AM, Ciccorossi P, Sacco R, Colombatto P, et al. Transient elastography: A new surrogate marker of liver fibrosis influenced by major changes of transaminases. Journal of Viral Hepatitis. 2007;**14**(5):360-369. DOI: 10.1111/j.1365-2893.2006.00811.x

[63] Sagir A, Erhardt A, Schmitt M, Häussinger D. Transient elastography is unreliable for detection of cirrhosis in patients with acute liver damage. Hepatology. 2008;**47**(2):592-595. DOI: 10.1002/hep.22056

[64] Arena U, Vizzutti F, Corti G, Ambu S, Stasi C, Bresci S, et al. Acute viral hepatitis increases liver stiffness values measured by transient elastography. Hepatology. 2008;**47**(2): 380-384. DOI: 10.1002/hep.22007

[65] Millonig G, Reimann FM, Friedrich S, Fonouni H, Mehrabi A, Büchler MW, et al. Extrahepatic cholestasis increases liver stiffness (FibroScan) irrespective of fibrosis. Hepatology. 2008;**48**(5):1718-1723. DOI: 10.1002/hep.22577

[66] Millonig G, Friedrich S, Adolf S, Fonouni H, Golriz M, Mehrabi A, et al. Liver stiffness is directly influenced by central venous pressure. Journal of Hepatology. 2010;**52**(2): 206-210. DOI: 10.1016/j.jhep.2009.11.018

[67] Petta S, Maida M, Macaluso FS, Di Marco V, Cammà C, Cabibi D, et al. The severity of steatosis influences liver stiffness measurement in patients with nonalcoholic fatty liver disease. Hepatology. 2015;**62**(4):1101-1110. DOI: 10.1002/hep.27844

[68] Lupșor-Platon M, Feier D, Stefănescu H, Tamas A, Botan E, Sparchez Z, et al. Diagnostic accuracy of controlled attenuation parameter measured by transient elastography for the non-invasive assessment of liver steatosis: A prospective study. Journal of Gastrointestinal and Liver Diseases. 2015;**24**:35-42. DOI: 10.15403/jgld.2014.1121.mlp

[69] Wang Y, Fan Q, Wang T, Wen J, Wang H, Zhang T. Controlled attenuation parameter for assessment of hepatic steatosis grades: A diagnostic meta-analysis. International Journal of Clinical and Experimental Medicine 2015;**8**(10):17654-17663. eCollection 2015

[70] Shi KQ, Tang JZ, Zhu XL, Ying L, Li DW, Gao J, et al. Controlled attenuation parameter for the detection of steatosis severity in chronic liver disease: A meta-analysis of diagnostic accuracy. Journal of Gastroenterology and Hepatology. 2014;**29**:1149-1158. DOI: 10.1111/jgh.12519

[71] de Lédinghen V, Vergniol J, Foucher J, Merrouche W, le Bail B. Non-invasive diagnosis of liver steatosis using controlled attenuation parameter (CAP) and transient elastography. Liver International. 2012;**32**:911-918. DOI: 10.1111/j.1478-3231.2012.02820.x

[72] Kumar M, Rastogi A, Singh T, Behari C, Gupta E, Garg H, et al. Controlled attenuation parameter for noninvasive assessment of hepatic steatosis: Does etiology affect performance? Journal of Gastroenterology and Hepatology. 2013;**28**:1194-1201. DOI: 10.1111/jgh.12134

[73] Shen F, Zheng RD, Mi YQ, Wang XY, Pan Q, Chen GY, et al. Controlled attenuation parameter for non-invasive assessment of hepatic steatosis in Chinese patients. World Journal of Gastroenterology. 2014;**20**:4702-4711. DOI: 10.3748/wjg.v20.i16.4702

[74] Chan WK, Nik Mustapha NR, Mahadeva S. Controlled attenuation parameter for the detection and quantification of hepatic steatosis in nonalcoholic fatty liver disease. Journal of Gastroenterology and Hepatology. 2014;**29**:1470-1476. DOI: 10.1111/jgh.12557

[75] de Lédinghen V, Vergniol J, Capdepont M, Chermak F, Hiriart JB, Cassinotto C, et al. Controlled attenuation parameter (CAP) for the diagnosis of steatosis: A prospective

study of 5323 examinations. Journal of Hepatology. 2014;**60**:1026-1031. DOI: 10.1016/j.jhep.2013.12.018

[76] Myers RP, Pollett A, Kirsch R, Pomier-Layrargues G, Beaton M, Levstik M, et al. Controlled attenuation parameter (CAP): A noninvasive method for the detection of hepatic steatosis based on transient elastography. Liver International. 2012;**32**:902-910. DOI: 10.1111/j.1478-3231.2012.02781.x

[77] Karlas T, Petroff D, Sasso M, Fan JG, Mi YQ, de Lédinghen V, et al. Individual patient data meta-analysis of controlled attenuation parameter (CAP) technology for assessing steatosis. Journal of Hepatology. 2017;**66**(5):1022-1030. DOI: 10.1016/j.jhep.2016.12.022

[78] Madsen EL, Sathoff HJ, Zagzebski JA. Ultrasonic shear wave properties of soft tissues and tissuelike materials. The Journal of the Acoustical Society of America. 1983;**74**:1346-1355

[79] Frizzell LA, Carstensen EL. Shear properties of mammalian tissues at low megahertz frequencies. The Journal of the Acoustical Society of America. 1976;**60**:1409-1411

[80] Lupsor M, Badea R, Stefanescu H, Sparchez Z, Branda H, Serban A, et al. Performance of a new elastographic method (ARFI technology) compared to unidimensional transient elastography in the noninvasive assessment of chronic hepatitis C. Preliminary results. Journal of Gastrointestinal and Liver Diseases. 2009;**18**(3):303-310

[81] Zhai L, Palmeri ML, Bouchard RR, Nightingale RW, Nightingale KR. An integrated indenter-ARFI imaging system for tissue stiffness quantification. Ultrasonic Imaging. 2008;**30**:95-111. DOI: 10.1177/016173460803000203

[82] Nightingale K, Soo MS, Nightingale R, Trahey G. Acoustic radiation force impulse imaging: In vivo demonstration of clinical feasibility. Ultrasound in Medicine & Biology. 2002;**28**:227-235. DOI: http://dx.doi.org/10.1016/S0301-5629(01)00499-9

[83] Mauldin FW Jr, Zhu HT, Behler RH, Nichols TC, Gallippi CM. Robust principal component analysis and clustering methods for automated classification of tissue response to ARFI excitation. Ultrasound in Medicine & Biology. 2008;**34**:309-325. DOI: 10.1016/j.ultrasmedbio.2007.07.019

[84] Fahey BJ, Nightingale KR, Nelson RC, Palmeri ML, Trahey GE. Acoustic radiation force impulse imaging of the abdomen: Demonstration of feasibility and utility. Ultrasound in Medicine & Biology. 2005;**31**:1185-1198. DOI: http://dx.doi.org/10.1016/j.ultrasmedbio.2005.05.004

[85] Bota S, Mare R, Sporea I. Point shear wave elastography. In: Sporea I, Sirli R, editors. Hepatic Elastography Using Ultrasound Waves. Revised edition of volume 1. Sharjah, UAE: Bentham Science Publishers; 2016. pp. 44-87. DOI: 10.2174/97816080546331120101

[86] Bota S, Herkner H, Sporea I, Salzl P, Sirli R, Neghina AM, et al. Meta-analysis: ARFI elastography versus transient elastography for the evaluation of liver fibrosis. Liver International. 2013;**33**(8):1138-1147. DOI: 10.1111/liv.12240

[87] Popescu A, Sporea I, Sirli R, Bota S, Focşa M, Dănilă M, et al. The mean values of liver stiffness assessed by acoustic radiation force impulse elastography in normal subjects. Medical Ultrasonography. 2011;**13**(1):33-37

[88] Son CY, Kim SU, Han WK, Choi GH, Park H, Yang SC, et al. Normal liver elasticity values using acoustic radiation force impulse imaging: A prospective study in healthy living liver and kidney donors. Journal of Gastroenterology and Hepatology. 2012;**27**(1): 130-136. DOI: 10.1111/j.1440-1746.2011.06814.x

[89] Madhok R, Tapasvi C, Prasad U, Gupta AK, Aggarwal A. Acoustic radiation force impulse imaging of the liver: Measurement of the normal mean values of the shearing wave velocity in a healthy liver. Journal of Clinical and Diagnostic Research. 2013;**7**(1): 39-42. DOI: 10.7860/JCDR/2012/5070.2665

[90] Popescu A, Bota S, Sporea I, Sirli R, Danila M, Racean S, et al. The influence of food intake on liver stiffness values assessed by acoustic radiation force impulse elastography-preliminary results. Ultrasound in Medicine & Biology. 2013;**39**(4):579-584. DOI: 10.1016/j.ultrasmedbio.2012.11.013

[91] Bota S, Sporea I, Peck-Radosavljevic M, Sirli R, Tanaka H, Iijima H, et al. The influence of aminotransferase levels on liver stiffness assessed by acoustic radiation force impulse elastography: A retrospective multicentre study. Digestive and Liver Disease. 2013;**45**(9):762-768. DOI: 10.1016/j.dld.2013.02.008

[92] Fierbinteanu Braticevici C, Sporea I, Panaitescu E, Tribus L. Value of acoustic radiation force impulse imaging elastography for non-invasive evaluation of patients with nonalcoholic fatty liver disease. Ultrasound in Medicine & Biology. 2013;**39**(11):1942-1950. DOI: 10.1016/j.ultrasmedbio.2013.04.019

[93] Cassinotto C, Lapuyade B, Aït-Ali A, Vergniol J, Gaye D, Foucher J, et al. Liver fibrosis: Noninvasive assessment with acoustic radiation force impulse elastography—Comparison with FibroScan M and XL probes and FibroTest in patients with chronic liver disease. Radiology. 2013;**269**(1):283-292. DOI: 10.1148/radiol.13122208

[94] Friedrich-Rust M, Romen D, Vermehren J, Kriener S, Sadet D, Herrmann E, et al. Acoustic radiation force impulse-imaging and transient elastography for non-invasive assessment of liver fibrosis and steatosis in NAFLD. European Journal of Radiology. 2012;**81**(3):e325-ee31. DOI: 10.1016/j.ejrad.2011.10.029

[95] Guzmán-Aroca F, Frutos-Bernal M, Bas A, Luján-Mompeán J, Reus M, de Dios Berná-Serna J, et al. Detection of non-alcoholic steatohepatitis in patients with morbid obesity before bariatric surgery: Preliminary evaluation with acoustic radiation force impulse imaging. European Radiology. 2012;**22**(11):2525-2532. DOI: 10.1007/s00330-012-2505-3

[96] Osaki A, Kubota T, Suda T, Igarashi M, Nagasaki K, Tsuchiya A, et al. Shear wave velocity is a useful marker for managing nonalcoholic steatohepatitis. World Journal of Gastroenterology. 2010;**16**(23):2918-2925. DOI: 10.3748/wjg.v16.i23.2918

[97] Palmeri ML, Wang MH, Rouze NC, Abdelmalek MF, Guy CD, Moser B, et al. Noninvasive evaluation of hepatic fibrosis using acoustic radiation force-based shear stiffness in patients with nonalcoholic fatty liver disease. Journal of Hepatology. 2011;**55**(3):666-672. DOI: 10.1016/j.jhep.2010.12.019

[98] Yoneda M, Suzuki K, Kato S, Fujita K, Nozaki Y, Hosono K, et al. Nonalcoholic fatty liver disease: US-based acoustic radiation force impulse elastography. Radiology. 2010;**256**(2):640-647. DOI: 10.1148/radiol.10091662

[99] Liu H, Fu J, Hong R, Liu L, Li F. Acoustic radiation force impulse elastography for the non-invasive evaluation of hepatic fibrosis in non-alcoholic fatty liver disease patients: A systematic review & meta-analysis. PLoS One. 2015;**10**(7):e0127782. DOI: 10.1371/journal.pone.0127782. eCollection 2015

[100] Muller M, Gennisson JL, Deffieux T, Tanter M, Fink M. Quantitative viscoelasticity mapping of human liver using supersonic shear imaging: Preliminary in vivo feasibility study. Ultrasound in Medicine & Biology. 2009;**35**(2):219-229. DOI: 10.1016/j.ultrasmedbio.2008.08.018

[101] Ferraioli G, Tinelli C, Zicchetti M, Above E, Poma G, Di Gregorio M, et al. Reproducibility of real-time shear wave elastography in the evaluation of liver elasticity. European Journal of Radiology. 2012;**81**:3102-3106. DOI: 10.1016/j.ejrad.2012.05.030

[102] Kudo M, Shiina T, Moriyasu F, Iijima H, Tateishi R, Yada N, et al. JSUM ultrasound elastography practice guidelines: Liver. Journal of Medical Ultrasonics. 2013;**40**:325-357. DOI: 10.1007/s10396-013-0460-5

[103] Lupşor-Platon M, Badea R, Gersak M, Maniu A, Rusu I, Suciu A, et al. Noninvasive assessment of liver diseases using 2D shear wave elastography. Journal of Gastrointestinal and Liver Diseases. 2016;**25**(4):525-532. DOI: http://dx.doi.org/10.15403/jgld.2014.1121.254.lup

[104] Leung VY, Shen J, Wong VW, Abrigo J, Wong GL, Chim AM, et al. Quantitative elastography of liver fibrosis and spleen stiffness in chronic hepatitis B carriers: Comparison of shear-wave elastography and transient elastography with liver biopsy correlation. Radiology. 2013 Dec;**269**(3):910-918. DOI: 10.1148/radiol.13130128

[105] Suh CH, Kim SY, Kim KW, Lim YS, Lee SJ, Lee MG, et al. Determination of normal hepatic elasticity by using real-time shear-wave elastography. Radiology. 2014;**271**(3):895-900. DOI: 10.1148/radiol.14131251

[106] Procopet B, Berzigotti A, Abraldes JG, Turon F, Hernandez-Gea V, García-Pagán JC, et al. Real-time shear-wave elastography: Applicability, reliability and accuracy for clinically significant portal hypertension. Journal of Hepatology. 2015;**62**:1068-1075. DOI: 10.1016/j.jhep.2014.12.007

[107] Ferraioli G, Tinelli C, Dal Bello B, Zicchetti M, Filice G, Filice C, Liver Fibrosis Study Group. Accuracy of real-time shear wave elastography for assessing liver fibrosis in chronic hepatitis C: A pilot study. Hepatology. 2012;**56**:2125-2133. DOI: 10.1002/hep.25936

[108] Bavu E, Gennisson JL, Couade M, Bercoff J, Mallet V, Fink M, et al. Noninvasive in vivo liver fibrosis evaluation using supersonic shear imaging: A clinical study on 113 hepatitis C virus patients. Ultrasound in Medicine & Biology. 2011;**37**(9):1361-1373. DOI: 10.1016/j.ultrasmedbio.2011.05.016

[109] Yoon JH, Lee JY, Woo HS, Yu MH, Lee ES, Joo I, et al. Shear wave elastography in the evaluation of rejection or recurrent hepatitis after liver transplantation. European Radiology. 2013;**23**(6):1729-1737. DOI: 10.1007/s00330-012-2748-z

[110] Sporea I, Bota S, Jurchis A, Sirli R, Grădinaru-Tascău O, Popescu A, et al. Acoustic radiation force impulse and supersonic shear imaging versus transient elastography for liver fibrosis assessment. Ultrasound in Medicine & Biology. 2013;**39**(11):1933-1941. DOI: 10.1016/j.ultrasmedbio.2013.05.003

[111] Cassinotto C, Lapuyade B, Mouries A, Hiriart JB, Vergniol J, Gaye D, et al. Non-invasive assessment of liver fibrosis with impulse elastography: Comparison of supersonic shear imaging with ARFI and FibroScan®. Journal of Hepatology. 2014;**61**:550-557. DOI: 10.1016/j.jhep.2014.04.044

[112] Jiang T, Tian G, Zhao Q, Kong D, Cheng C, Zhong L, et al. Diagnostic accuracy of 2D-shear wave elastography for liver fibrosis severity: A meta-analysis. PLoS One. 2016;**11**:e0157219. DOI: 10.1371/journal.pone.0157219

[113] Li C, Zhang C, Li J, Huo H, Song D. Diagnostic accuracy of real-time shear wave elastography for staging of liver fibrosis: A meta-analysis. Medical Science Monitor. 2016;**22**:1349-1359. DOI: 10.12659/MSM.895662

Section 2

Prevention and Treatment

Chapter 6

Management of Nonalcoholic Fatty Liver Disease (NAFLD)

Monjur Ahmed

Additional information is available at the end of the chapter

http://dx.doi.org/10.5772/intechopen.72000

Abstract

Although there is an epidemic of NAFLD throughout the world, the management of NAFLD is not very satisfactory at the present time. Lifestyle modification is the main mode of therapy. Other modalities like pharmacotherapy and bariatric endoscopy or surgery should be individualized. Various pharmacological agents are being investigated to optimize the treatment of NAFLD.

Keywords: nonalcoholic fatty liver disease, fatty liver, hepatic steatosis, nonalcoholic steatohepatitis, NASH, treatment of NAFLD

1. Introduction

When we consider the management of Nonalcoholic Fatty Liver Disease (NAFLD), two aspects should be considered. One is that it can be a part of the metabolic syndrome [1]. About 80% of patients with metabolic syndrome have NAFLD [2]. Although the prevalence of NAFLD is 20–40% in the general population, about 70% of type 2 diabetes mellitus [3] and 85% of patients with morbid obesity (BMI ≥ 40) have NAFLD [4]. In the general population, 80% of patients with NAFLD are overweight and 20% of NAFLD patients have normal weight as per ultrasonography [5]. Another aspect is that it covers a spectrum of hepatic involvement as it progresses slowly from one stage to another. Initially, it starts as simple steatosis or benign fatty liver disease or nonalcoholic fatty liver (NAFL), where there is only macrovesicular hepatic steatosis (>5% of hepatocytes are affected) without any inflammation, hepatocellular injury or fibrosis [6]. The second phase is nonalcoholic steatohepatitis (NASH) where there is not only hepatic steatosis but also ballooning degeneration of hepatocytes and mixed inflammatory cells (lymphocytes, plasma cells, monocytes, neutrophils and eosinophils) infiltrates mainly involving the hepatic acini [7]. The third phase is hepatic fibrosis which generally starts from zone 3 and progresses to bridging fibrosis, cirrhosis of liver and hepatocellular cancer. Prognosis depends on the degree of liver fibrosis [8].

2. Purpose

The main purpose of management of NAFLD is to halt the process as soon as it is diagnosed. The three main modalities of therapy include lifestyle modification, pharmacotherapy and bariatric surgery. Lifestyle modification is applicable to all stages of NAFLD, whereas pharmacotherapy and bariatric surgery should not be considered for patients with simple steatosis. Pharmacotherapy should be considered only for patients with biopsy-proven NASH and hepatic fibrosis as per the guideline of American Association for the Study of Liver Diseases (AASLD).

3. Lifestyle modification

As NAFLD is related to insulin resistance, gradual weight loss is extremely important in overweight and obese individuals [9]. Rapid weight loss can cause portal inflammation and fibrosis [10]. About 7–10% of weight loss over one year by lifestyle changes has been associated with histological improvement in simple steatosis and NASH [11]. Another study showed vigorous and moderate exercises were equally effective in reducing hepatic triglyceride content largely through weight loss [12]. Diet and moderate aerobic exercise are the first line measures to reduce weight and improve insulin resistance [13]. Dietary counseling should be highly encouraged. Consumption of high fructose containing food is the main cause of epidemic of obesity [14]. Patient should avoid high fructose containing foods like sweet, soda, desserts, breakfast cereals, granola bars and cakes. One study showed that in patients with NAFLD, fructokinase and fatty acid synthase activity are increased [15]. NAFLD may occur when there is a combination of genetic predisposition, sedentary life style and consumption of high-calorie foods [16]. One meta-analysis suggested that Omega-3 fatty acid supplementation in diet was beneficial in patients with NAFLD/NASH [17]. Patients should be encouraged to eat food rich in Omega-3 fatty acid (fish, canola, olive, perilla and chia). Food with high glycemic effects and saturated fat should be avoided [18].

In summary, lifestyle modification is the first line intervention in the management of NAFLD. This includes [1] weight loss of about 7–10% of body weight by a combination of diet and exercise [2], low-calorie diet [3], diet with high fructose and saturated fat should be avoided [4], diet with Omega-3 fatty acid supplement should be encouraged.

4. Pharmacotherapy

There are various pharmacological agents available for the management of NAFLD. Many of them have been found to be ineffective and some of them have high risk-benefit ratio [19]. There are various clinical trials ongoing. Here, we discuss the common agents available and the agents recommended by the American Association for the Study of Liver Diseases (ASSLD).

4.1. Antioxidants

Progression of simple steatosis to steatohepatitis is related to oxidative stress and free radical formation. Vitamin E has been studied in different clinical trials. One study showed that patients with vitamin E deficiency and NAFLD did not respond to the classical diet for NAFLD [20]. In PIVENS trial, vitamin E 800 units per day was associated with improvement of serum transaminases and liver histology in nondiabetic NAFLD patients [21]. Fibrosis scores were not improved in this trial [22]. In SELECT trial, vitamin E supplementation 400 units per day in healthy individuals was associated with significant increase in prostate cancer [23].

Currently, vitamin E 800 units per day is recommended in nondiabetic individuals with biopsy-proven NASH [19].

4.2. Insulin sensitizing agents

4.2.1. Thioglitazones (TZD)

They are agonists/selective ligands of nuclear transcription factor PPAR-ϒ (peroxisome proliferator-activated receptor-gamma) which is present in pancreatic β-cells, adipocytes, skeletal muscles, endothelial cells and macrophages. They increase insulin sensitivity in NAFLD and thus, promote fatty acid transportation from liver and skeletal muscles into adipose tissue, decrease serum-free fatty acid concentration and increase fatty acid oxidation in the liver [24]. Pioglitazone 30 mg/day improved hepatic steatosis, steatohepatitis and transaminitis in nondiabetic patients with NASH in the PIVENS trial but histological response did not reach statistical significance [22]. Another study showed that in prediabetic and diabetic patients, long-term treatment with pioglitazone 45 mg/day improved not only steatotic and inflammatory activity but also hepatic fibrosis [25]. There are few concerns about the side effects of TZD and these include weight gain [26], bone loss [27] and congestive heart failure [28].

As pioglitazone improves histology of NASH in both diabetic and nondiabetic individuals, it can be used in biopsy-proven NASH. Patients should be informed about the efficacy and side effects of this medication.

4.2.2. Incretin-based therapy

Glucagon-like peptide 1 (GLP-1) receptor agonists (liraglutide and exenatide) not only improves insulin sensitivity but also causes weight loss by suppressing appetite and inhibiting gastric emptying [29]. They are primarily used to control diabetes mellitus at this time. There are case reports of improvement of hepatic steatosis by GLP-1 receptor agonists [30]. Another study found that liraglutide given daily improved steatohepatitis and decreased progression of fibrosis [31].

Although incretin mimetics have been found to be helpful in diabetic patients with NAFLD, they are currently not recommended solely to treat NASH or NAFLD [19].

4.2.3. Bariatric surgery

As sustained weight loss is achievable by bariatric surgery, all the features of metabolic syndrome improve and there is reduction in mortality [32]. In a prospective study, NASH disappeared in 70% (severe NASH) to 94% (mild NASH) of patients 1 year after bariatric surgery [33]. There are various bariatric surgical and endoscopic procedures available and approved for morbid obesity at the present time. Laparoscopic sleeve gastrectomy is most commonly done in the United States [34]. Other surgical procedures include gastric bypass, biliointestinal bypass, biliopancreatic diversion with duodenal switch, vertical band gastroplasty and gastric banding. Various endoscopic procedures include intragastric balloon placement, endoscopic sleeve gastroplasty [35] and duodenal mucosal resurfacing [36]. Bariatric endoscopy is successful in reducing more weight than pharmacological agents but less effective than bariatric surgery but has less complications than bariatric surgery. Bower et al. found in a systematic review of studies that bariatric surgery improved steatosis, steatohepatitis and fibrosis in NAFLD [37]. Patients with cirrhosis of liver due to NAFLD are at a higher risk for bariatric surgery [38]. Another study showed that perioperative mortality was higher in patients with NAFLD with cirrhosis than in patients with NAFLD without cirrhosis [39].

Nowadays, bariatric surgery is not recommended as a primary treatment of NAFLD but it can be considered in obese individuals with noncirrhotic NAFLD [19].

4.2.4. Ursodeoxycholic acid (UDCA)

UDCA has cytoprotective effect and can improve serum transaminases in NAFLD but cannot alter liver histology [40].

UDCA is not recommended for the treatment of NAFLD or NASH [19].

4.2.5. Omega-3 fatty acids

Although in animal models, omega-3 fatty acid treatment improved hepatic steatosis [41, 42], recent studies did not show any significant effect on serum transaminases or liver histology [43]. Omega-3 fatty acid is not recommended for the treatment of NAFLD or NASH.

4.2.6. Obeticholic acid (OCA)

OCA is a ligand of farnesoid X receptor (FXR) which is a nuclear receptor present in liver, kidneys, intestine and adipose tissue. FXR controls target genes involved in bile acid synthesis and transport as well as lipid and carbohydrate metabolism. In the farnesoid X receptor ligand obeticholic acid in NASH treatment (FLINT) trial, OCA induced weight loss and improved hepatic fibrosis but resolution of NASH was not statistically more than placebo. OCA decreased serum transaminases but increased serum alkaline phosphatase, LDL and blood glucose levels [44].

Currently, OCA is not recommended in the routine management of NAFLD awaiting the completion of phase 3 trial (REGENERATE) of OCA for the treatment of NASH patients with liver fibrosis [45].

http://dx.doi.org/10.5772/intechopen.72000

5. Elafibranor

Elafibranor is an agonist of PPAR-α and δ receptor. It has anti-inflammatory activity and can improve insulin sensitivity and lipid metabolism. It was evaluated in a phase II international study for the treatment of NASH [46]. In the post hoc analysis, elafibranor (120 mg/day for 1 year) group showed resolution of NASH without progression of fibrosis more than placebo (19% vs. 12%).

As the improvement was marginal, further studies are needed before using this agent in the treatment of NAFLD.

5.1. Statins

Hyperlipidemia is frequently seen in patients with NAFLD as part of the metabolic syndrome. Statins are commonly used for the treatment of hyperlipidemia, and low-to-moderate dose of statins have been found to be safe with low hepatic toxicity [47]. Statins decrease hepatic transaminases and hepatic fat but have no effect on hepatic fibrosis [48, 49].

Statins are not currently recommended solely for the treatment of NAFLD unless the patient has concomitant hyperlipidemia.

5.2. Orlistat

Orlistat is used as a weight reducing agent as it induces fat malabsorption by inhibiting enteric and pancreatic lipase [50]. A randomized controlled trial showed that orlistat improved transaminitis and hepatitis steatosis in obese individuals with NAFLD [51]. Subsequent study suggested that orlistat did not have any direct effect on NAFLD, overweight subjects improved their hepatic histology if they achieved ≥5% weight loss irrespective of taking orlistat [52].

Currently, orlistat cannot be recommended primarily for NAFLD.

5.3. NAFLD and cirrhosis

Patients should be managed the same way as in other cirrhosis. Patients with NAFLD-cirrhosis have 2.6% annual cumulative risk of developing hepatocellular cancer [53]. For every 6 months, abdominal ultrasound is recommended for screening of hepatocellular carcinoma. In obese individuals, if ultrasound is technically difficult, CT or MRI should be considered. As obesity and hyperinsulinemia are risk factors for malignancy, liver cancer can occur even in noncirrhotic NAFLD [54]. Screening for esophageal and gastric varices should be done at base-line of diagnosis of cirrhosis and at regular intervals—no varices: every 2–3 years, small varices—every 1–2 years and decompensated cirrhosis—yearly once [55].

With the epidemic of NAFLD, NASH-cirrhosis and hepatocellular carcinoma will be the leading indication of liver transplantation in future. As patients with NAFLD have multiple metabolic and cardiovascular comorbidities, they should be managed posttransplant appropriately. Management of NAFLD involves multiple specialties which include primary care physicians, gastroenterologists, hepatologists, endocrinologists, bariatric surgeons, transplant surgeons, dietitians and nutritionists.

6. Future therapy

As hepatic inflammation, fibrosis, cirrhosis and subsequent malignancy are the main concerns of NAFLD, plenty of research and studies on anti-inflammatory and anti-fibrotic agents are on-going.

7. Summary

The management of NAFLD patients should be individualized (**Table 1**).

- Lifestyle change is the first line therapy: healthy food habit, increased physical activity, exercise and weight loss of 7–10%.
- Pharmacotherapy is to be considered when lifestyle changes fail to achieve the goal: vitamin E in nondiabetic biopsy-proven NASH, pioglitazone in both diabetic and nondiabetic biopsy-proven NASH, incretin mimetics in diabetes mellitus and NAFLD, statins in hyperlipidemia and NAFLD, orlistat in NAFLD and obesity when life-style changes fail to reduce weight loss.
- Bariatric surgery should be considered in obese individuals and noncirrhotic NAFLD.

Lifestyle changes	First line therapy of NAFLD
Vitamin E	Nondiabetic biopsy-proven NASH
Pioglitazone	Both diabetic and nondiabetic biopsy-proven NASH
Incretin mimetics	Diabetes mellitus and NAFLD
Statins	Hyperlipidemia and NAFLD
Orlistat	NAFLD and obesity when lifestyle changes fail
Bariatric surgery	Morbid obesity and noncirrhotic NAFLD

Table 1. Summary of management of NAFLD.

Author details

Monjur Ahmed

Address all correspondence to: monjur.ahmed@jefferson.edu

Thomas Jefferson University, Philadelphia, PA, USA

References

[1] Lonardo A, Ballestri S, Marchesini G, Angulo P, Loria P. Nonalcoholic fatty liver disease: A precursor of the metabolic syndrome. Digestive and Liver Disease. 2015;**47**(3):181-190. DOI: 10.1016/j.dld.2014.09.020 Epub 2014 Nov 18

[2] Antunes C, Bhimji S. Fatty Liver. StatPearls [Internet]. Treasure Island (FL): StatPearls Publishing; 2017. PMID: 28723021

[3] Leite NC, Salles GF, Araujo AL, Villela-Nogueira CA, Cardoso CR. Prevalence and associated factors of non-alcoholic fatty liver disease in patients with type-2 diabetes mellitus. Liver International. 2009;**29**(1):113-119. DOI: 10.1111/j.1478-3231.2008.01718.x Epub 2008 Apr 1

[4] Fabbrini E, Sullivan S, Klein S. Obesity and Nonalcoholic Fatty Liver Disease: Biochemical, Metabolic and Clinical Implications. Hepatology. 2010;**51**(2):679-689. DOI: 10.1002/hep.23280

[5] Bellentani S, Tiribelli C. The spectrum of liver disease in the general population: Lesson from the Dionysos study. Journal of Hepatology. 2001;**35**(4):531-537 PMID: 11682041

[6] Contos MJ, Sanyal AJ. The clinicopathologic spectrum and management of nonalcoholic fatty liver disease. Advances in Anatomic Pathology. 2002;**9**(1):37-51 PMID: 11756758

[7] Harmon RC, Tiniakos DG, Argo CK. Inflammation in nonalcoholic steatohepatitis. Expert Review of Gastroenterology and Hepatology. 2011;**5**(2):189-200. DOI: 10.1586/egh.11.21

[8] Angulo P, Machado MV, Diehl AM. Fibrosis in nonalcoholic Fatty liver disease: Mechanisms and clinical implications. Seminars in Liver Disease. 2015;**35**(2):132-145. DOI: 10.1055/s-0035-1550065 Epub 2015 May 14

[9] Harrison SA, Day CP. Benefits of lifestyle modification in NAFLD. Gut. 2007;**56**(12):1760-1769. DOI: 10.1136/gut.2006.112094 PMCID: PMC2095707

[10] Andersen T, Gluud C, Franzmann MB, Christoffersen P. Hepatic effects of dietary weight loss in morbidly obese subjects. Journal of Hepatology. 1991;**12**(2):224-229 PMID: 2051001

[11] Tilg H, Moschen A. Weight loss: Cornerstone in the treatment of non-alcoholic fatty liver disease. Minerva Gastroenterologica e Dietologica. 2010;**56**(2):159-167

[12] Zhang HJ, He J, Pan LL, Ma ZM, Han CK, Chen CS, Chen Z, Han HW, Chen S, Sun Q, Zhang JF, Li ZB, Yang SY, Li XJ, Li XY. Effects of moderate and vigorous exercise on nonalcoholic fatty liver disease: A randomized clinical trial. JAMA Internal Medicine. 2016;**176**(8):1074-1082. DOI: 10.1001/jamainternmed.2016.3202

[13] Wilkins T, Tadkod A, Hepburn I, Schade RR. Nonalcoholic fatty liver disease: Diagnosis and management. American Family Physician. 2013;**88**(1):35-42

[14] Bray GA, Nielson SJ, Popkin BM. Consumption of high-fructose corn syrup in beverages may play a role in the epidemic of obesity. American Journal of Clinical Nutrition. 2004;**79**(4):537-543

[15] Ouyang X, Cirillo P, Sautin Y, McCall S, Bruchette JL, Diehl AM, Johnson RJ, Abdelmalek MF. Fructose consumption as a risk factor for non-alcoholic fatty liver disease. Journal of Hepatology. 2008;**48**(6):993-999. DOI: 10.1016/j.jhep.2008.02.011 Epub 2008 Mar 10

[16] Dongiovanni P, Romeo S, Valenti L. Genetic factors in the pathogenesis of nonalcoholic fatty liver and steatohepatitis. Biomed Research International. 2015;**2015**:460190. DOI: 10.1155/2015/460190 Epub 2015 Jul 27. PMID: 26273621. PMCID: PMC4530215

[17] Lu W, Li S, Li J, Wang J, Zhang R, Zhou Y, Yin Q, Zheng Y, Wang F, Xia Y, Chen K, Liu T, Lu J, Zhou Y, Guo C. Effects of omega-3 fatty acid in nonalcoholic fatty liver disease: A meta-analysis. Gastroenterology Research and Practice. 2016;**2016**:1459790. DOI: 10.1155/2016/1459790 PMCID: PMC5019889

[18] Ferolla SM, Silva LC, Ferrari MDLA, Cunha ASD, Martins FDS, Couto CA, Ferrari TCA. Dietary approach in the treatment of nonalcoholic fatty liver disease. World Journal of Hepatology. 2015;**7**(24):2522-2534. DOI: 10.4254/wjh.v7.i24.2522 PMCID: PMC4621466

[19] Chalasani N, Younossi Z, Lavine JE, Charlton M, Cusi K, Rinella M, Harrison SA, Brunt EM, Sanyal AJ. The diagnosis and management of nonalcoholic fatty liver disease: Practice guidance from the American Association for the Study of Liver Diseases. Hepatology. 2017. DOI: 10.1002/hep.29367 [Epub ahead of print]. PMID: 28714183

[20] Cankurtaran M, Kav T, Yavuz B, Shorbagi A, Halil M, Coskun T, Arslan S. Serum vitamin-E levels and its relation to clinical features in nonalcoholic fatty liver disease with elevated ALT levels. Acta Gastro-enterologica Belgica. 2006;**69**(1):5-11

[21] Chalasani NP, Sanyal AJ, Kowdley KV, Robuck PR, Hoofnagle J, Kleiner DE, Unalp A, Tonascia J, NASH CRN Research Group. Pioglitazone versus vitamin E versus placebo for the treatment of non-diabetic patients with non-alcoholic steatohepatitis: PIVENS trial design. Contemporary Clinical Trials. 2009;**30**(1):88-96. DOI: 10.1016/j.cct.2008.09.003 Epub 2008 Sep 10

[22] Sanyal AJ, Chalasani N, Kowdley KV, McCullough A, Diehl AM, Bass NM, Neuschwander-Tetri BA, Lavine JE, Tonascia J, Unalp A, Van Natta M, Clark J, Brunt EM, Kleiner DE, Hoofnagle JH, Robuck PR, NASH CRN. Pioglitazone, vitamin E, or placebo for nonalcoholic steatohepatitis. New England Journal of Medicine. 2010;**362**(18):1675-1685. DOI: 10.1056/NEJMoa0907929 Epub 2010 Apr 28

[23] Klein EA, Thompson IM Jr, Tangen CM, Crowley JJ, Lucia MS, Goodman PJ, Minasian LM, Ford LG, Parnes HL, Gaziano JM, Karp DD, Lieber MM, Walther PJ, Klotz L, Parsons JK, Chin JL, Darke AK, Lippman SM, Goodman GE, Meyskens FL Jr, Baker LH. Vitamin E and the risk of prostate cancer: The Selenium and Vitamin E Cancer Prevention Trial (SELECT). Journal of the American Medical Association. 2011;**306**(14):1549-1556. DOI: 10.1001/jama.2011.1437

[24] Mehta SR. Advances in the treatment of nonalcoholic fatty liver disease. Therapeutic Advances in Endocrinology and Metabolism. 2010;**1**(3):101-115. DOI: 10.1177/2042018810379587 PMCID: PMC3475281

[25] Cusi K, Orsak B, Bril F, Lomonaco R, Hecht J, Ortiz-Lopez C, Tio F, Hardies J, Darland C, Musi N, Webb A, Portillo-Sanchez P. Long-term pioglitazone treatment for patients with nonalcoholic steatohepatitis and prediabetes or type 2 diabetes mellitus: A randomized trial. Annals of Internal Medicine. 2016;**165**(5):305-315. DOI: 10.7326/M15-1774 Epub 2016 Jun 21. PMID: 27322798

[26] Aghamohammadzadeh N, Niafar M, Dalir Abdolahinia E, et al. The effect of pioglitazone on weight, lipid profile and liver enzymes in type 2 diabetic patients. Therapeutic Advances in Endocrinology and Metabolism. 2015;**6**(2):56-60. DOI: 10.1177/2042018815574229

[27] Lecka-Czernik B. Bone loss in diabetes: Use of antidiabetic thiazolidinediones and secondary osteoporosis. Current Osteoporosis Reports. 2010;**8**(4):178-184. DOI: 10.1007/s11914-010-0027 PMID: 20809203

[28] Jearath V, Vashisht R, Rustagi V, Raina S, Sharma R. Pioglitazone-induced congestive heart failure and pulmonary edema in a patient with preserved ejection fraction. Journal of Pharmacology & Pharmacotherapeutics. 2016;**7**(1):41-43. DOI: 10.4103/0976-500X.179363

[29] Prasad-Reddy L, Isaacs D. A clinical review of GLP-1 receptor agonists: Efficacy and safety in diabetes and beyond. Drugs Context. 2015;**4**:212283. DOI: 10.7573/dic.212283 PMCID: PMC4509428

[30] Tushuizen ME, Bunck MC, Pouwels PJ, van Waesberghe JH, Diamant M, Heine RJ. Incretin mimetics as a novel therapeutic option for hepatic steatosis. Liver International. 2006;**26**(8):1015-1017. DOI: 10.1111/j.1478-3231.2006.01315.x 16953843

[31] Armstrong MJ, Gaunt P, Aithal GP, Barton D, Hull D, Parker R, Hazlehurst JM, Guo K, LEAN trial team, Abouda G, Aldersley MA, Stocken D, Gough SC, Tomlinson JW, Brown RM, Hübscher SG, Newsome PN. Liraglutide safety and efficacy in patients with non-alcoholicsteatohepatitis (LEAN): A multicentre, double-blind, randomised, placebo-controlled phase 2 study. Lancet. 2016;**387**(10019):679-690. DOI: 10.1016/S0140-6736(15)00803-X Epub 2015 Nov 20

[32] Adams TD, Gress RE, Smith SC, Halverson RC, Simper SC, Rosamond WD, Lamonte MJ, Stroup AM, Hunt SC. Long-term mortality after gastric bypass surgery. New England Journal of Medicine. 2007;**357**(8):753-761 PMID: 17715409

[33] Lassailly G, Caiazzo R, Buob D, Pigeyre M, Verkindt H, Labreuche J, Raverdy V, Leteurtre E, Dharancy S, Louvet A, Romon M, Duhamel A, Pattou F, Mathurin P. Bariatric surgery reduces features of nonalcoholic steatohepatitis in morbidly obese patients. Gastroenterology. 2015;**149**(2):379-388; quiz e15-6. DOI: 10.1053/j.gastro.2015.04.014 Epub 2015 Apr 25

[34] Donatelli G, Dumont JL, Cereatti F, Ferretti S, Vergeau BM, Tuszynski T, Pourcher G, Tranchart H, Mariani P, Meduri A, Catheline JM, Dagher I, Fiocca F, Marmuse JP, Meduri B. Treatment of leaks following sleeve gastrectomy by endoscopic internal drainage (EID). Obesity Surgery. 2015;**25**(7):1293-1301. DOI: 10.1007/s11695-015-1675-x PMID: 25913755

[35] Choi HS, Chun HJ. Recent trends in endoscopic bariatric therapies. Clinical Endoscopy. 2017;**50**(1):11-16. DOI: 10.5946/ce.2017.007

[36] Cherrington AD, Rajagopalan H, Maggs D, Devière J. Hydrothermal duodenal mucosal resurfacing: Role in the treatment of metabolic disease. Gastrointestinal Endoscopy Clinic of North America. 2017;**27**(2):299-311. DOI: 10.1016/j.giec.2016.12.002

[37] Bower G, Toma T, Harling L, Jiao LR, Efthimiou E, Darzi A, Athanasiou T, Ashrafian H. Bariatric surgery and non-alcoholic fatty liver disease: A systematic review of liver biochemistry and histology. Obesity Surgery. 2015;**25**(12):2280-2289. DOI: 10.1007/s11695-015-1691-x

[38] Grimm IS, Schindler W, Haluszka O. Steatohepatitis and fatal hepatic failure after biliopancreatic diversion. American Journal of Gastroenterology. 1992;**87**(6):775-779 PMID: 1590319

[39] Mosko JD, Nguyen GC. Increased perioperative mortality following bariatric surgery among patients with cirrhosis. Clinical Gastroenterology and Hepatology. 2011;**9**(10):897-901. DOI: 10.1016/j.cgh.2011.07.007 Epub 2011 Jul 23

[40] Lindor KD, Kowdley KV, Heathcote EJ, Harrison ME, Jorgensen R, Angulo P, Lymp JF, Burgart L, Colin P. Ursodeoxycholic acid for treatment of nonalcoholic steatohepatitis: Results of a randomized trial. Hepatology. 2004;**39**(3):770-778. DOI: 10.1002/hep.20092 PMID: 14999696

[41] Di Minno MND, Russolillo A, Lupoli R, Ambrosino P, Di Minno A, Tarantino G. Omega-3 fatty acids for the treatment of non-alcoholic fatty liver disease. World Journal of Gastroenterology: WJG. 2012;**18**(41):5839-5847. DOI: 10.3748/wjg.v18.i41.5839

[42] Scorletti E, Bhatia L, McCormick KG, Clough GF, Nash K, Hodson L, Moyses HE, Calder PC, Byrne CD, WELCOME Study. Effects of purified eicosapentaenoic and docosahexaenoic acids in nonalcoholic fatty liver disease: Results from the Welcome* study. Hepatology. 2014;**60**(4):1211-1221. DOI: 10.1002/hep.27289 PMID: 25043514

[43] Sanyal AJ, Abdelmalek MF, Suzuki A, Cummings OW, Chojkier M, EPE-A Study Group. No significant effects of ethyl-eicosapentanoic acid on histologic features of nonalcoholic steatohepatitis in a phase 2 trial. Gastroenterology. 2014;**147**(2):377-84.e1. DOI: 10.1053/j.gastro.2014.04.046 Epub 2014 May 9

[44] Makri E, Cholongitas E, Tziomalos K. Emerging role of obeticholic acid in the management of nonalcoholic fatty liver disease. World Journal of Gastroenterology. 2016;**22**(41):9039-9043. DOI: 10.3748/wjg.v22.i41.9039

[45] Randomized Global Phase 3 Study to Evaluate the Impact on NASH With Fibrosis of Obeticholic Acid Treatment (REGENERATE). https://clinicaltrials.gov/ct2/show/NCT02548351

[46] Ratziu V, Harrison SA, Francque S, Bedossa P, Lehert P, Serfaty L, Romero-Gomez M, Boursier J, Abdelmalek M, Caldwell S, Drenth J, Anstee QM, Hum D, Hanf R, Roudot A, Megnien S, Staels B, Sanyal A, GOLDEN-505 Investigator Study Group. Elafibranor, an agonist of the peroxisome proliferator-activated receptor-α and δ, induces resolution of nonalcoholic steatohepatitis without fibrosis worsening. Gastroenterology. 2016;**150**(5):1147-1159.e5. DOI: 10.1053/j.gastro.2016.01.038 Epub 2016 Feb 11

[47] Athyros VG, Mikhailidis DP, Didangelos TP, Giouleme OI, Liberopoulos EN, Karagiannis A, Kakafika AI, Tziomalos K, Burroughs AK, Elisaf MS. Effect of multifactorial treatment on non-alcoholic fatty liver disease in metabolic syndrome: A randomised study. Current Medical Research and Opinion. 2006;**22**(5):873-883

[48] Lowyck I, Fevery J. Statins in hepatobiliary diseases: Effects, indications and risks. Acta Gastro-enterologica Belgica. 2007;**70**(4):381-388 18330098

[49] Eslami L, Merat S, Malekzadeh R, Nasseri-Moghaddam S, Aramin H. Statins for non-alcoholic fatty liver disease and non-alcoholic steatohepatitis. Cochrane Database of Systematic Reviews. 2013;**12**:CD008623. DOI: 10.1002/14651858.CD008623.pub2

[50] Guerciolini R. International Journal of Obesity and Related Metabolic Disorders: Journal of the International Association for the Study of Obesity. 1997;**21**(Supplement 3):S12-S23

[51] Zelber-Sagi S, Kessler A, Brazowsky E, Webb M, Lurie Y, Santo M, Leshno M, Blendis L, Halpern Z, Oren R. A double-blind randomized placebo-controlled trial of orlistat for the treatment of nonalcoholic fatty liver disease. Clinical Gastroenterology and Hepatology. 2006;**4**(5):639-644 Epub 2006 Apr 17

[52] Harrison SA, Fecht W, Brunt EM, Neuschwander-Tetri BA. Orlistat for overweight subjects with nonalcoholic steatohepatitis: A randomized, prospective trial. Hepatology. 2009;**49**(1):80-86. DOI: 10.1002/hep.22575

[53] Ascha MS, Hanouneh IA, Lopez R, Tamimi TA, Feldstein AF, Zein NN. The incidence and risk factors of hepatocellular carcinoma in patients with nonalcoholic steatohepatitis. Hepatology. 2010;**51**(6):1972-1978. DOI: 10.1002/hep.23527

[54] Kawada N, Imanaka K, Kawaguchi T, Tamai C, Ishihara R, Matsunaga T, Gotoh K, Yamada T, Tomita Y. Hepatocellular carcinoma arising from non-cirrhotic nonalcoholic steatohepatitis. Journal of Gastroenterology. 2009;**44**(12):1190-1194. DOI: 10.1007/s00535-009-0112-0

[55] Garcia-Tsao G, Sanyal AJ, Grace ND, Carey W. Practice Guidelines Committee of the American Association for the Study of Liver Diseases; Practice Parameters Committee of the American College of Gastroenterology. Prevention and management of gastroesophageal varices and variceal hemorrhage in cirrhosis. Hepatology. 2007;**46**(3):922-938. DOI: 10.1002/hep.21907 PMID: 17879356

Chapter 7

Nutrition and Lifestyle Modifications in the Prevention and Treatment of Non-Alcoholic Fatty Liver Disease

Kingsley Asare Kwadwo Pereko, Jacob Setorglo,
Matilda Steiner-Asiedu and
Joyce Bayebanona Maaweh Tiweh

Additional information is available at the end of the chapter

http://dx.doi.org/10.5772/intechopen.71368

Abstract

Non-alcoholic fatty liver disease (NAFLD) is a burgeoning health problem worldwide. NAFLD is an umbrella term for a range of liver conditions affecting people who drink little to no alcohol Different methods are employed in the diagnosis of NAFLD. Certain drugs, genetics, lifestyle factors have been implicated in the development of NAFLD. NAFLD symptoms are asymptomatic but indicated when there is unexplained persistent elevation of liver enzyme levels. Nutrition and lifestyle modifications are widely prescribed as helpful in the prevention and treatment of Non-Alcoholic Fatty Liver disease (NAFLD). Dietary and lifestyle modifications are apparent measures considering the disease association with obesity, diabetes, and cardiovascular disease which many reviews have linked to the condition. Reduction in body weight, involvement in both aerobic and anaerobic exercises, conscious intake in the types of fat and carbohydrates are helpful in the management of NAFLD. This chapter highlights the various theories and principles underlying nutrition and lifestyle modifications in the prevention and treatment of NAFLDs.

Keywords: fatty liver, obesity, non-alcoholic, dietary, lifestyle

1. Introduction

Non-alcoholic fatty liver disease (NAFLD) is a burgeoning health problem worldwide and is a risk factor for both hepatic and cardiometabolic mortality [1, 2]. A meta-analysis of prevalence, incidence and outcome of NAFLD following publications on pubmed from 1989 to 2015 estimated global prevalence at 25.24% (95% CI: 22.10–28.65) with highest prevalence in the Middle East 31.79% (13.48–58.23) and South America 30.45% (22.74–39.44) and lowest in Africa 13.48% (5.69–28.69) [2]. NAFLD describes a range of conditions caused by a build-up of fat within liver cells and can be divided into four stages namely:

1. Simple fatty liver (hepatic steatosis). Under normal conditions, very little fat is stored in liver cells of humans. Hepatic steatosis therefore refers to a situation where excess fat accumulates in the hepatic cells. Sometimes simple fatty liver does not cause any harm to the liver or pose health risks. However, in some instances it leads to NAFLD and its severe forms and that is where the problem arises.
2. Non-alcoholic steatohepatitis (NASH). This expression is much less common than NAFLD. Here, the excess fat stored in the liver cells is associated with inflammation of the liver.
3. Fibrosis: This is associated with persistent hepatitis, including steatohepatitis and may lead to scarring of the liver tissue (fibrosis). This is not life threatening since when fibrosis some of the liver cells that continue to perform its functions.
4. Cirrhosis: This stage of a liver disease can be life threatening because normal liver tissues are replaced by a lot of fibrosis. The structure and function of the liver are therefore modified. There are different scientific means of detecting liver diseases.

2. Diagnosis

There are different methods of diagnosing NAFLD. The test ranges from metabolic syndrome assessment, detecting metabolites in the blood as well as enzymes such as Alanine transaminase (ALT) and Aspartate Aminotransferase (AST) [3]. Medical imaging and sonographic techniques are also performed to create an image of the liver. Further tests such as fibroscan and biopsy may be conducted apart from those listed earlier to determine the stage of the liver disease [4].

3. Risk factors

A wide range of diseases and conditions can predispose one to non-alcoholic fatty liver disease (NAFLD). Non-alcoholic steatohepatitis expresses itself among some sub-populations such as older people, diabetics and the obese. Certain drugs and hepatitis have been implicated in the development of NAFLD as well. Some risks are usually from lifestyle origin. These include:

- High cholesterol and triglycerides levels,
- Metabolic syndrome,

- Central adiposity,
- Polycystic ovary syndrome,
- Sleep apnea,
- Genetics,
- Hypothyroidism,
- Hypopituitarism [5].

Nutritional factors have also been cited as risks in the development of the disease. These include rapid weight loss, total parenteral nutrition, starvation and protein-calorie malnutrition [6]. The most common risk factor associated with NAFLD is the presence of the metabolic syndrome. The metabolic syndrome is defined by the presence of 3 or more of the following criteria (**Table 1**): (1) increased waist circumference, (2) hypertriglyceridemia, (3) hypertension, (4) high fasting glucose, and (5) a low high-density lipoprotein (HDL) level.

Parameter*	Value
Impaired glucose tolerance	Fasting blood glucose level ≥ 110 mg/dL
High blood pressure	≥130/85 mm Hg
Elevated triglyceride levels	>250 mg/dL
Low high-density lipoprotein level	<40 mg/dL for men; <50 mg/dL for women
Abdominal obesity	Waist: >102 cm (40 inches) for men; >88 cm (35 inches) for women

*Metabolic syndrome is diagnosed by the presence of 2 or more of these parameters.
Source: [2].

Table 1. Diagnostic criteria for metabolic syndrome.

4. Signs and symptoms and management

Nonalcoholic fatty liver disease occurs in every age group but especially in people in their 40s and 50s. The condition is also closely linked to metabolic syndrome, which is a cluster of abnormalities including increased abdominal fat, poor ability to use the hormone insulin, high blood pressure and high blood levels of triglycerides. NAFLD symptoms are asymptomatic but indicated when there is unexplained persistent elevation of liver enzyme levels after hepatitis and other chronic liver diseases have been excluded. However, at certain stages of the disease, patients are malaise, fatigue, and right upper quadrant or diffuse abdominal discomfort. Hepatomegaly is found on clinical examination. When there is cirrhosis there may be; spider angiomata, ascites, splenomegaly, hard liver border, ascites, portal hypertension and jaundice or pruritus [7].

Clinical evaluation includes a careful history and physical examination. It is relevant to inquire about excess alcohol consumption which is defined as intakes greater than 30 g/day for men and greater than 20 g/day for women within the past 5 years. A drink is 350 mL (12 oz) of beer, 120 mL (4 oz) of wine, and 45 mL (1.5 oz) of hard liquor each contain 10 g of alcohol.

There are several approaches to managing NAFLD. Hepatoprotective therapy, antioxidants insulin-sensitizing agents and treatment of obesity are part of these. However, this text limits itself to the nutritional management of the NAFLD. Key to nutritional therapeutic procedures are lifestyle changes in diet and improving exercise habits in addition to the control of comorbidities which are secondary to the development of NAFLD [8]. For instance, bile acid derivatives and associated compounds that influence bile acid related are becoming prominent therapeutic agents for NAFLD [9, 10, 11]. The immediate associated lifestyle causes of NAFLD are targeted in the management of the disease condition.

5. Obesity and genetics

Obesity when combined with physical inactivity and genetic predisposition, has been directly associated with metabolic syndrome and NAFLD among some adult populations [12, 2]. Obesity itself is the failure of normal homeostatic regulation of energy utilization [9]. NAFLD can be a precursor to developing metabolic syndrome or insulin resistance [10]. Data suggest that about 80% of adults who are class 1 and/or 2 obese and 90% morbid obese according to the World Health Organization classification are at risk of having NAFLD [13]. Body weight loss can alter the cellular activity of adipose tissue and reverse many of the negative consequences of NAFLD. The excess fat and energy content of a meal has been associated with NAFLD development in healthy populations [14, 15]. Insulin resistance, oxidative stress, and cytokine toxicity results due to obesity and these factors have been implicated in the pathogenesis of NAFLD [16]. Among these factors, central adiposity and insulin resistance have direct association with hepatic fat content and visceral adiposity [17–19]. Polymorphisms (genetic variations) in the single-nucleotide polymorphisms (SNPs) T455C and C482T in APOC3 are associated with fatty liver disease. The carriers of T-455C, C-482 T, or both (not additive) had a 30% increase in fasting plasma apolipoprotein C3, 60% increase in fasting plasma triglyceride and 46% reduction in plasma triglyceride clearance. Oxidative stress, hormonal imbalances, and mitochondrial abnormalities can be potential causes.

6. Total fat

Dietary composition of a meal in terms of the macro-molecule distribution has a positive relation with the development of NAFLD. The amount and type of dietary fat may directly affect liver fat content, with high-fat diets being potentially harmful [20]. It has also been shown that a high ratio of omega-6 to omega-3 polyunsaturated fatty acids (PUFAs) and an increased intake of saturated and trans fatty acids are associated with NAFLD [21–23]. It was noted that when severely obese patients were fed diets containing higher percentage of total fat beyond recommended ranges, the risk of developing NALFD increased [24]. The deduction therefore was that the type of fat ingested rather than the amount is associated with NAFLD in obese individuals.

7. Saturated fatty acids

Saturated fatty acid component in meals has been shown to induce insulin resistance especially among the obese [25–27]. In epidemiologic studies, both total fat and saturated fat in the diet had significant correlation with triglyceride content in hepatic cells [28, 29]. In a double-blind randomized controlled trial of two reduced-fat diets, compared with a control diet both reduced-fat diets decreased amount of low density lipoprotein cholesterol (LDLc) in healthy males [30]. There was a decrease in high density lipoprotein cholesterol (HDLc) and increase in triglyceride levels increased with the reduced-fat diets. The authors concluded that reduced saturated fat intake (below 10%) may benefit patients with NAFLD. It was also observed that, low total fat and low saturated fat diet (23% fat and 7% saturated fat) predicted changes in HDLc and LDLc but not the amount of fat in the hepatocytes [31].

8. *Trans* fatty acids

Trans fatty acids are positively associated with an increase in inflammatory processes, plasma triglycerides, and cholesterol as well as a reduction in HDLc level [32, 33]. Animal studies have shown positive relationships between the increased consumption of trans fatty acids from oxidized oils and liver inflammation [34, 35].

9. Polyunsaturated fatty acids (PUFAs)

Essential fatty acid, Omega-3 (which is a type of polyunsaturated fatty acids) PUFA levels are decreased in the hepatic tissue of people with NAFLD [22, 36] A higher omega-6 to omega-3 PUFA ratio may contribute to the development of a fatty liver within the hepatocytes of people NAFLD [36].

10. High carbohydrate intake

High carbohydrate intake especially the amount and type of carbohydrate consumed have an important impact on the development of NAFLD [37]. Simple carbohydrates intakes can lead to the development of NAFLD [38]. Meals high in carbohydrates lead to increased amounts of circulating insulin, which contribute to elevated triglyceride concentrations even under isocaloric conditions [39, 40]. A higher carbohydrate intake more than the recommended daily values has been positively associated with liver inflammation and NAFLD [24].

Coupled with a low-fat meal, high-carbohydrate meal promotes the development of a NAFLD through increased de novo fatty acid and triglyceride synthesis [41].

11. High-fructose corn syrup intake

Epidemiological data suggest that dietary pattern and an increased intake of simple sugars, especially fructose is associated with the development of NAFLD [42, 43]. The link is not too clear although it is assumed that the carbohydrates components increased risk of fatty infiltration of the liver or muscle. Therefore it was hypothesized that the link is through both indirect and direct mechanisms [44, 45]. Indirect association manifest itself through the adverse metabolic effects that can increase the risk of developing NAFLD. Fructose may cause hepatotoxic damage as a form of direct route link with NAFLD. Studies [46–49] have suggested that increased fructose consumption augments fat mass, de novo lipogenesis, and inflammation. There is also induction of insulin resistance and fasting and postprandial triglycerides, which in turn, can result in liver steatosis. In other studies [50, 51], sugar-sweetened beverage consumption was found to be associated with fatty liver independent of body mass index of the individuals. Direct positive association was found between the amount of fructose consumed and the development of NAFLD [52, 53]. Age and frequency of consuming fructose-based food was also found to be related to liver inflammation and NAFLD [54].

12. Physical inactivity

Physical activity has been documented to improve health and hence the World Health Organization recommendations for aerobic an anaerobic exercises across the life span. Physical inactivity however, has been associated with NAFLD. Using matched controls for age and gender, only about one-fifth of individuals with NAFLD met recommendations for physical activity [55, 56]. Among 349 individuals studied, the NAFLD group engaged in less physical activity, including total, aerobic, and resistance [55].

It has been noted that decreased physical activity correlates with intra-hepatic fat, decreased cellular insulin sensitivity, and increased central adiposity [57, 58]. Sedentary time alone is associated with metabolic status. Sedentary times predicted higher levels of fasting insulin, independent of the amount of time spent engaging in moderate- or vigorous-intensity activity [59]. Therefore to improve metabolic health it is generally important to reduce sedentary lifestyle even when one meets the requirements for physical activity.

13. Treatments

Aggressive pursuit of modified lifestyle modifications coupled with dietary changes are critical in treating NAFLD when body weight is the underlying cause. That is because dietary macronutrient composition, physical activity, and all play critical roles in successful weight reduction. Weight loss is effective for improving NAFLD as it positively influences insulin sensitivity and dyslipidemia.

14. Body weight loss

It was found that about 9% body weight loss significantly improves NAFLD [60]. The result was thought to be due to improvements in inflammation and steatosis. Reduction in body weight through lowering of daily caloric intake of about 200 kcal/day improved liver cellular structure histology and enzymes function. A 10% body weight reduction resulted in a 45% reduction in liver fat content [61]. Lifestyle modification through dietary intake, exercise, and behavior modification with the guidelines from health experts has been show to lead to resolution in NALFD [62]. A weight reduction of about 7% was therefore recommended [63]. A combination of diet and exercise reduces fibrosis and amount of liver fat by an average of 40% [64–66]. The degree of hepatic fat reduction is related to the intensity of the lifestyle mediation and normally required a weight loss range of 5–10% is suggested.

15. Bariatric surgery

Among persons with higher grades of obesity, physical remedy such as reduction in dietary intake and physical activities does not result in resolution of NAFLD. Other means such as bariatric surgery is the most effective strategy to achieve and maintain weight loss [67]. Results from several uncontrolled studies [68–70] and controlled studies [71, 72] indicated that body weight loss achieved through bariatric surgery reduces amount of liver enzymes and improves NAFLD.

A study found an association between bariatric surgery and lower serum alanine transferase and aspartate aminotransferase levels at two and 10 years follow-up [73] and histological improvements [74]. Steatosis, steatohepatitis, and fibrosis improved among majority of patients that have undergone surgery [75]. It is worth noting that hepatic decompensation can occur after gastric bypass so decision to opt for this should be taken with great care [3].

16. Nutrient content and healthful fats

Dietary composition can directly manipulate NAFLD progress. Changing either the composition of the macronutrient or micronutrient content can directly affect the level of inflammation, amount of serum lipids and insulin resistance [49]. Inverse association was found between Mediterranean diet consumption and cardiovascular disease risk [76]. Among obese women and overweight men, a low-fat diet decreased hepatic fat compared with a high-fat diet [64, 77]. The dietary recommendation is that the diet contain less than 7% saturated fats, less than 1% of trans fats and 25–35% of the calorific intake should be total fat among which is polyunsaturated fatty acid.

17. Monounsaturated fats

It was found that replacing carbohydrate intake with monounsaturated fatty acids (MUFAs) to about 32 g/day increases triglyceride-rich lipoprotein catabolism [30]. This can lead to resolution of NAFLD. This finding is supported by epidemiological studies [31, 78]. Olive oil which contains about 73% MUFAs appears to provide a direct benefit in improving plasma lipids and possible NAFLD [79]. In randomized trials, [80, 81] isocaloric low-fat/high-carbohydrate diet improved hepatic fat and improved insulin sensitivity. The diet was composed of 50% MUFAs and 18% omega-3 PUFAs, 40% from carbohydrate, and 20% protein. These findings were independent of body weight loss of patients.

18. Omega-3 Omega-6 PUFAs

Evidence from epidemiologic and randomized controlled trials indicate that supplementation with omega-3 PUFAs lowers triglyceride levels and reduces the risk of coronary heart disease and mortality.94,95 High consumption of omega-3 PUFAs derived from fish diminishes hepatic triglyceride lipoprotein secretion and inhibits de novo lipogenesis. [82]. Using the Therapeutic Lifestyle Change diet criteria with a diet high in fish-derived omega-3 fatty acid (1.23 g/day EPA + DHA) vs. a low fish diet (0.27 g/day EPA + DHA) for 24 weeks, the higher fish diet decreased plasma triglycerides by 24%. Three human clinical trials support these findings by showing that giving patients with NAFLD omega-3 PUFAs (1 to 2.7 g/day for six to 12 months) improved hepatic steatosis, inflammation, and fibrosis [82, 83]. Capanni and Spadaro both demonstrated that triglyceride levels decreased 25 to 37 mg/dL when patients' diets were supplemented with 1 to 2 g of omega-3 PUFAs per day for six and 12 months, respectively. This was thought to be through diminishes hepatic triglyceride lipoprotein secretion and inhibition de novo lipogenesis [82–84]. Diets based on therapeutic lifestyle change criteria supports improvements in NAFLD as the diet improves liver steatosis, inflammation, and fibrosis [85]. In a non-controlled trial, omega-6 PUFAs (15% of energy as linoleic acid) reduced liver fat compared with a diet high in saturated fatty acids in abdominally obese patients [86]. A diet consisting of mainly reduced simple carbohydrate may confer similar benefits among NALFD patients [87, 88].

19. Low sugar intake

Diet designed to produce a caloric deficit of 500 to1000 kcal/day is advised. Reduction of dietary carbohydrates, in particular dietary fructose, is the most beneficial and has been found to improve the lipid profile in overweight patients. Diets with less carbohydrate and more fat have relatively greater benefits in NAFLD management [89, 90]. Hypocaloric diet made up from 40% carbohydrate and 45% fat decreased serum alanine transaminase concentration than did a higher-carbohydrate (60%), low-fat diet (25% fat) [91]. Low-carbohydrate caloric restriction significantly improved hepatic insulin sensitivity. Diets with less carbohydrate and more fat have relatively greater benefits for insulin levels, triglycerides, and HDL cholesterol concentrations than do hypocaloric, low-fat diets. A hypocaloric diet moderately lower in carbohydrate (40% carbohydrate and 45% fat) decreased serum alanine transaminase concentrations to a greater degree than did a higher-carbohydrate, low-fat diet (60% carbohydrate and 25% fat).106 For individuals with NAFLD who were glucose intolerant, the low-carbohydrate caloric restriction significantly improved hepatic insulin sensitivity compared with the low-fat diet. In contrast, changes in visceral fat mass and insulin sensitivity were similar between a low-calorie, reduced-carbohydrate diet (fewer than 90 g of carbohydrate) and a reduced-fat diet (less than 20% fat). The World Health Organization recommends that the daily intake of added sugars makes up no more than 10% of total energy. The American Heart Association recommends limiting the amount of added sugars to no more than one-half of daily discretionary calories, which for women is approximately 100 kcal/day (6 tsp. of sugar) and for men is 150 kcal/day (9 tsp. of sugar).

20. Physical activity therapy

Physical activity enhances insulin sensitivity and favorably modifies lipids independent of weight loss [92, 93] Data suggest that there is improvement in cellular liver characteristics when NALFD individuals become active [94]. Exercise can lead to improvement in insulin sensitivity which intends contributes to the fatty acid delivery to the liver [95]. Improvement in insulin resistance and may decrease hepatic steatosis, inflammation, and disease progression in NAFLD [96, 97]. Four studies have investigated the effects of exercise without dietary modification on hepatic steatosis. Exercise can independently results in reduction in the fat in the hepatocytes without a significant weight change [98–101].

21. Exercise intensity and duration

Both intermittent and daily exercise helps achieve weight loss and improve insulin sensitivity [102]. Intensity and duration contribute to energy expenditure and therefore can lead to insulin sensitivity, triglycerides, and serum glucose amount [103]. Vigorous exercise and doubling the duration of vigorous exercise was associated with decreased odds of developing fat in the liver [104]. Increased exercise by 60 minutes or more per week significantly reduced body weight and all liver enzymes [105]. Regular aerobic exercise for half an hour at least per day at 60–70% max heart rate for least 5 days per week reduces liver alanine transaminase levels [106].

22. Aerobic and resistance exercises

Increased aerobic exercise has been associated with improvement in the metabolic parameters associated with NAFLD [61, 94, 106]. Combined aerobic and resistance exercises have been shown to be more effective than aerobic exercise alone for resolving inflammation and cardio-vascular risk factors [107]. An intervention of 30 minutes of aerobic exercise and 20 minutes of resistance exercise three times per week was found to be associated with improvements in hepatic fat among NAFLD patients [108]. This combination activity improves hepatic insulin sensitivity [100] reduction in liver fat [109]. Both findings were independent of body weight reduction. Antioxidant treatments such as vitamins and minerals supplementation have been mentioned to decrease oxidative stress and improve oxidative injury among NAFLD patients.

23. Vitamin E

In theory, vitamin E and other vitamins called antioxidants could help protect the liver by reducing or neutralizing the damage caused by inflammation. But more research is needed. Some evidence suggests vitamin E supplements may be helpful for people with liver damage caused by nonalcoholic fatty liver disease [110]. But vitamin E has been linked with increased risk of death and, in men, an increased risk of prostate cancer. Several small trials in humans with NAFLD have supported an effect of tocopherol (vitamin E) on the improvement of trans-aminase levels but there have been discordant results in histologic improvement [111]. There was a significant improvement in hepatic steatosis with vitamin E intakes at levels of 800 to 1000 IU/day [112, 113] Higher intakes of the vitamin can be fatal in most cases [114, 115].

24. Vitamin D

Vitamin D may play an important role in modifying the risk of cardio metabolic outcomes [116, 117]. Serum 25-hydroxy vitamin D concentrations were correlated with NAFLD in terms of liver steatosis, inflammation and fibrosis [118].

25. EPA + DHA

The evidence supporting the use of omega-3 PUFAs for treating NAFLD have consisted of small sample sizes and laden with errors [118, 119].

26. Probiotics

Gut microbiota has been associated with the development of obesity-related NAFLD [120]. Probiotics may improve liver enzymes and decrease markers of lipid peroxidation [121, 122]. The use of prebiotics and probiotics is to modify the microbiota as preventive or therapeutic strategies [123]. Their beneficial effects on NAFLD have been limited human studies [124]. Consuming a tablet containing 500 million *Lactobacillus bulgaricus* and *Streptococcus thermophilus* for 3 months improved levels of liver enzyme in patients with NAFLD [124].

27. Other nutrients

Ginger (*Zingiber officinale*) can improve insulin sensitivity and reduce hepatic fat content [125]. In studies of people with non-alcoholic fatty liver disease, those who reported drinking coffee had less liver damage than those who drank little or no coffee. It's not clear how coffee may influence liver damage or how much coffee you'd need to drink in order to benefit. **Table 2** summarizes the nutritional guidelines in the management and treatment of NAFLD.

Weight loss	10% of initial body weight over 6 months Maintenance of weight loss Bariatric surgery when individuals qualify
Calorie intake	1200 to 1500 daily **Energy deficit of 500 kcal/day based on Mifflin-St Jeor formula*
Total fat	≤ 35% of total calories
Monounsaturated fatty acids	15–25% of total calories
Polyunsaturated fatty acids	5–10% of total calories Omega-3 fatty acids
Saturated fatty acids	7–10% of total calories
Carbohydrate	50% of total calories > 50% carbohydrate sources from whole grains Avoid high-fructose corn syrup Added sugars <10% of total calories
Protein	15% of total calories Lean and vegetable protein
Antioxidants	None
Physical activity	≥ 150 minutes/week at moderate intensity or ≥75 minutes/week at vigorous intensity Cardiovascular exercise five times weekly Resistance training two or more times weekly Decrease time spent sedentary

Source: [65, 81, 83].

Table 2. Guidelines in the management and treatment of NAFLD.

Author details

Kingsley Asare Kwadwo Pereko[1]*, Jacob Setorglo[2], Matilda Steiner-Asiedu[3] and Joyce Bayebanona Maaweh Tiweh[4]

*Address all correspondence to: kpereko@gmail.com

1 School of Medical Sciences, University of Cape Coast, Cape Coast, Ghana

2 School of Allied Health Sciences, University of Cape Coast, Cape Coast, Ghana

3 Department of Nutrition and Food Science, University of Ghana, Legon, Ghana

4 Eye Unit, Manhyia Government Hospital, Kumasi, Ghana

References

[1] McCulough AJ. The clinical features, diagnosis and natural history of nonalcoholic fatty liver disease. Clinics in Liver Disease. Aug 2004;**8**(3):521-533. DOI: 10.1016/j.cld.2004.04.004. PMID 15331061

[2] Chalasani N, Younossi Z, Lavine JE, et al. The diagnosis and management of non-alcoholic fatty liver disease: Practice guideline by the American Association for the Study of Liver Diseases, American College of Gastroenterology, and the American Gastroenterological Association. Hepatology. 2012;**55**(6):2005-2023

[3] Chalasani N et al. The diagnosis and management of non-alcoholic fatty liver disease: Practice guideline by the American Association for the Study of Liver Diseases, American College of Gastroenterology, and the American Gastroenterological Association. American Journal of Gastroenterology. 2012;**107**(6):811-826

[4] Brunt EM. Pathology of non-alcoholic fatty liver disease. Nature Reviews. Gastroenterology & Hepatology. 2010;(4):195-203. Epub 2010 Mar 2

[5] Rinella ME. Nonalcoholic fatty liver disease: A systematic review. JAMA (Systematic Review). 2015;**313**(22):2263-2273. DOI: 10.1001/jama.2015.5370. PMID 26057287

[6] Allocca M, Selmi C. Emerging nutritional treatments for nonalcoholic fatty liver disease. In: Preedy VR, Lakshman R, Rajaskanthan RS, editors. Nutrition, Diet Therapy, and the Liver. Florida, USA: CRC Press; 2010. pp. 131-146. ISBN 1420085492

[7] Clark JM, Diehl AM. Nonalcoholic fatty liver disease: An underrecognized cause of cryptogenic cirrhosis. Journal of the American Medical Association. 2003;**289**(22):3000-3004. DOI: 10.1001/jama.289.22.3000. PMID 12799409

[8] Loria P, Adinolfi LE, Bellentani S, et al. Practice guidelines for the diagnosis and management of nonalcoholic fatty liver disease. A decalogue from the Italian Association for the study of the liver (AISF) expert committee. Digestive and Liver Disease. 2010;**42**(4):272-282

[9] Dandona P, Aljada A, Bandyopadhyay A. Inflammation: The link between insulin resistance, obesity and diabetes. Trends in Immunology. 2004;**25**(1):4-7

[10] Vanni E, Bugianesi E, Kotronen A, De Minicis S, Yki-Järvinen H, Svegliati-Baroni G. From the metabolic syndrome to NAFLD or vice versa? Digestive and Liver Disease. 2010;**42**(5):320-330

[11] Capristo E, Miele L, Forgione A, et al. Nutritional aspects in patients with non-alcoholic steatohepatitis (NASH). European Review for Medical and Pharmacological Sciences. 2005;**9**(5):265-268

[12] Marchesini G, Bugianesi E, Forlani G, et al. Nonalcoholic fatty liver, steatohepatitis, and the metabolic syndrome. Hepatology. 2003;**37**(4):917-923

[13] Gholam PM, Flancbaum L, Machan JT, Charney DA, Kotler DP. Nonalcoholic fatty liver disease in severely obese subjects. The American Journal of Gastroenterology. 2007;**102**(2):399-408

[14] Sobrecases H, Lê KA, Bortolotti M, et al. Effects of short-term overfeeding with fructose, fat and fructose plus fat on plasma and hepatic lipids in healthy men. Diabetes & Metabolism. 2010;**36**(3):244-246

[15] Ngo Sock ET, Le KA, Ith M, Kreis R, Boesch C, Tappy L. Effects of a short-term overfeeding with fructose or glucose in healthy young males. The British Journal of Nutrition. 2010;**103**(7):939-943

[16] Dowman JK, Tomlison JW, and Newsome PN. Pathogenesis of non-alcholic fatty liver disease. 2009;**103**:71-83 QJMed

[17] Jakobsen MU, Berentzen T, Sørensen TI, Overvad K. Abdominal obesity and fatty liver. Epidemiologic Reviews. 2007;**29**:77-87

[18] Chitturi S, Abeygunasekera S, Farrell GC, et al. NASH and insulin resistance: Insulin hypersecretion and specific association with the insulin resistance syndrome. Hepatol. 2002;**35**(2):373-379

[19] Lee JH, Rhee PL, Lee JK, et al. Role of hyperinsulinemia and glucose intolerance in the pathogenesis of nonalcoholic fatty liver in patients with normal body weight. The Korean Journal of Internal Medicine. 1998;**13**(1):12-14

[20] Donnelly KL, Smith CI, Schwarzenberg SJ, Jessurun J, Boldt MD, Parks EJ. Sources of fatty acids stored in liver and secreted via lipoproteins in patients with nonalcoholic fatty liver disease. The Journal of Clinical Investigation. 2005;**115**(5):1343-1351

[21] Kien CL. Dietary interventions for metabolic syndrome: Role of modifying dietary fats. Current Diabetes Reports. 2009;**9**(1):43-50

[22] Spadaro L, Magliocco O, Spampinato D, et al. Effects of n-3 polyunsaturated fatty acids in subjects with nonalcoholic fatty liver disease. Digestive and Liver Disease. 2008;**40**(3):194-199

[23] Tanaka N, Sano K, Horiuchi A, Tanaka E, Kiyosawa K, Aoyama T. Highly purified eicosapentaenoic acid treatment improves nonalcoholic steatohepatitis. Journal of Clinical Gastroenterology. 2008;**42**(4):413-418

[24] Solga S, Alkhuraishe AR, Clark JM, et al. Dietary composition and nonalcoholic fatty liver disease. Digestive Diseases and Sciences. 2004;**49**(10):1578-1583

[25] Lovejoy JC, Smith SR, Champagne CM, et al. Effects of diets enriched in saturated (palmitic), monounsaturated (oleic), or trans (elaidic) fatty acids on insulin sensitivity and substrate oxidation in healthy adults. Diabetes Care. 2002;**25**(8):1283-1288

[26] Vessby B, Uusitupa M, Hermansen K, et al. Substituting dietary saturated for monounsaturated fat impairs insulin sensitivity in healthy men and women: The KANWU study. Diabetologia. 2001;**44**(3):312-319

[27] Xiao C, Giacca A, Carpentier A, Lewis GF. Differential effects of monounsaturated, polyunsaturated and saturated fat ingestion on glucose-stimulated insulin secretion, sensitivity and clearance in overweight and obese, non-diabetic humans. Diabetologia. 2006;**49**(6):1371-1379

[28] Tiikkainen M, Bergholm R, Vehkavaara S, et al. Effects of identical weight loss on body composition and features of insulin resistance in obese women with high and low liver fat content. Diabetes. 2003;**52**(3):701-707

[29] Vilar L, Oliveira CP, Faintuch J, et al. High-fat diet: A trigger of non-alcoholic steatohepatitis? Preliminary findings in obese subjects. Nutrition. 2008;**24**(11-12):1097-1102

[30] Lefevre M, Champagne CM, Tulley RT, Rood JC. Most MM. Individual variability in cardiovascular disease risk factor responses to low-fat and low-saturated-fat diets in men: Body mass index, adiposity, and insulin resistance predict changes in LDL cholesterol. The American Journal of Clinical Nutrition. 2005;**82**(5):957-963

[31] Utzschneider KM, Bayer-Carter JL, Arbuckle MD, Tidwell JM, Richards TL, Craft S. Beneficial effect of a weight-stable, low-fat/low-saturated fat/low-glycaemic index diet to reduce liver fat in older subjects. The British Journal of Nutrition. 2013;**109**(6):1096-1104

[32] Eckel RH, Borra S, Lichtenstein AH, Yin-Piazza SY, Trans Fat Conference Planning Group. Understanding the complexity of trans fatty acid reduction in the American diet: American Heart Association trans fat conference 2006: Report of the trans fat conference planning group. Circulation. 2007;**115**(16):2231-2246

[33] Mensink RP, Zock PL, Kester AD, Katan MB. Effects of dietary fatty acids and carbohydrates on the ratio of serum total to HDL cholesterol and on serum lipids and apolipoproteins: A meta-analysis of 60 controlled trials. The American Journal of Clinical Nutrition. 2003;**77**(5):1146-1155

[34] Dhibi M, Brahmi F, Mnari A, et al. The intake of high fat diet with different trans fatty acid levels differentially induces oxidative stress and non alcoholic fatty liver disease (NAFLD) in rats. Nutrition & Metabolism (London). 2011;**8**(1):65

[35] Obara N, Fukushima K, Ueno Y, et al. Possible involvement and the mechanisms of excess trans-fatty acid consumption in severe NAFLD in mice. Journal of Hepatology. 2010;**53**(2):326-334

[36] Araya YN, Silvertown J, Gowing DJ, McConway KJ, Peter Linder H, Midgley G. A fundamental, eco-hydrological basis for niche segregation in plant communities. New Phytologist. 2011;**189**:253-258

[37] York LW, Puthalapattu S, Wu GY. Nonalcoholic fatty liver disease and low-carbohydrate diets. Annual Review of Nutrition. 2009;**29**:365-379

[38] Toshimitsu K, Matsuura B, Ohkubo I, et al. Dietary habits and nutrient intake in non-alcoholic steatohepatitis. Nutrition. 2007;**23**(1):46-52

[39] Garg A, Bantle JP, Henry RR, et al. Effects of varying carbohydrate content of diet in patients with non-insulin-dependent diabetes mellitus. Journal of the American Medical Association. 1994;**271**(18):1421-1428

[40] McLaughlin T, Abbasi F, Lamendola C, Yeni-Komshian H, Reaven G. Carbohydrate-induced hypertriglyceridemia: An insight into the link between plasma insulin and triglyceride concentrations. The Journal of Clinical Endocrinology and Metabolism. 2000;**85**(9):3085-3088

[41] Hudgins LC, Hellerstein M, Seidman C, Neese R, Diakun J, Hirsch J. Human fatty acid synthesis is stimulated by a eucaloric low fat, high carbohydrate diet. The Journal of Clinical Investigation. 1996;**97**(9):2081-2091

[42] Nomura K, Yamanouchi T. The role of fructose-enriched diets in mechanisms of nonalcoholic fatty liver disease. The Journal of Nutritional Biochemistry. 2012;**23**(3):203-208

[43] Alisi A, Manco M, Pezzullo M, Nobili V. Fructose at the center of necroinflammation and fibrosis in nonalcoholic steatohepatitis. Hepatology. 2011;**53**(1):372-373

[44] Lim JS, Mietus-Snyder M, Valente A, Schwarz JM, Lustig RH. The role of fructose in the pathogenesis of NAFLD and the metabolic syndrome. Nature Reviews. Gastroenterology & Hepatology. 2010;**7**(5):251-264

[45] Yilmaz Y. Review article: Fructose in non-alcoholic fatty liver disease. Alimentary Pharmacology & Therapeutics. 2012;**35**(10):1135-1144

[46] Huang D, Dhawan T, Young S, Yong WH, Boros LG, Heaney AP. Fructose impairs glucose-induced hepatic triglyceride synthesis. Lipids in Health and Disease. 2011;**10**:20

[47] Koo HY, Wallig MA, Chung BH, Nara TY, Cho BH, Nakamura MT. Dietary fructose induces a wide range of genes with distinct shift in carbohydrate and lipid metabolism in fed and fasted rat liver. Biochimica et Biophysica Acta. 2008;**1782**(5):341-348

[48] Teff KL, Elliott SS, Tschöp M, et al. Dietary fructose reduces circulating insulin and leptin, attenuates postprandial suppression of ghrelin, and increases triglycerides in women. The Journal of Clinical Endocrinology and Metabolism. 2004;**89**(6):2963-2972

[49] Stanhope KL, Havel PJ. Fructose consumption: Considerations for future research on its effects on adipose distribution, lipid metabolism, and insulin sensitivity in humans. The Journal of Nutrition. 2009;**139**(6):1236S-1241S

[50] Assy N, Nasser G, Kamayse I, et al. Soft drink consumption linked with fatty liver in the absence of traditional risk factors. Canadian Journal of Gastroenterology. 2008;**22**(10):811-816

[51] Abid A, Taha O, Nseir W, Farah R, Grosovski M, Assy N. Soft drink consumption is associated with fatty liver disease independent of metabolic syndrome. Journal of Hepatology. 2009;**51**(5):918-924

[52] Thuy S, Ladurner R, Volynets V, et al. Nonalcoholic fatty liver disease in humans is associated with increased plasma endotoxin and plasminogen activator inhibitor 1 concentrations and with fructose intake. The Journal of Nutrition. 2008;**138**(8):1452-1455

[53] Ouyang X, Cirillo P, Sautin Y, et al. Fructose consumption as a risk factor for non-alcoholic fatty liver disease. Journal of Hepatology. 2008;**48**(6):993-999

[54] Abdelmalek MF, Suzuki A, Guy C, et al. Increased fructose consumption is associated with fibrosis severity in patients with nonalcoholic fatty liver disease. Hepatology. 2010;**51**(6):1961-1971

[55] Zelber-Sagi S, Nitzan-Kaluski D, Goldsmith R, et al. Role of leisure-time physical activity in nonalcoholic fatty liver disease: A population-based study. Hepatology. 2008;**48**(6):1791-1798

[56] Krasnoff JB, Painter PL, Wallace JP, Bass NM, Merriman RB. Health-related fitness and physical activity in patients with nonalcoholic fatty liver disease. Hepatology. 2008;**47**(4):1158-1166

[57] Perseghin G, Lattuada G, De Cobelli F, et al. Habitual physical activity is associated with intrahepatic fat content in humans. Diabetes Care. 2007;**30**(3):683-688

[58] Booth FW, Laye MJ, Lees SJ, Rector RS, Thyfault JP. Reduced physical activity and risk of chronic disease: The biology behind the consequences. European Journal of Applied Physiology. 2008;**102**(4):381-390

[59] Helmerhorst HJ, Wijndaele K, Brage S, Wareham NJ, Ekelund U. Objectively measured sedentary time may predict insulin resistance independent of moderate- and vigorous-intensity physical activity. Diabetes. 2009;**58**(8):1776-1779

[60] Harrison SA, Fecht W, Brunt EM, Neuschwander-Tetri BA. Orlistat for overweight subjects with nonalcoholic steatohepatitis: A randomized, prospective trial. Hepatology. 2009;**49**(1):80-86

[61] Shah K, Stufflebam A, Hilton TN, Sinacore DR, Klein S, Villareal DT. Diet and exercise interventions reduce intrahepatic fat content and improve insulin sensitivity in obese older adults. Obesity (Silver Spring). 2009;**17**(12):2162-2168

[62] Promrat K, Kleiner DE, Niemeier HM, et al. Randomized controlled trial testing the effects of weight loss on nonalcoholic steatohepatitis. Hepatology. 2010;**51**(1):121-129

[63] Wong VW, Wong GL, Choi PC, et al. Disease progression of non-alcoholic fatty liver disease: A prospective study with paired liver biopsies at 3 years. Gut. 2010;**59**(7):969-974

[64] Westerbacka J, Lammi K, Häkkinen AM, et al. Dietary fat content modifies liver fat in overweight nondiabetic subjects. The Journal of Clinical Endocrinology and Metabolism. 2005;**90**(5):2804-2809

[65] Petersen KF, Dufour S, Befroy D, Lehrke M, Hendler RE, Shulman GI. Reversal of nonalcoholic hepatic steatosis, hepatic insulin resistance, and hyperglycemia by moderate weight reduction in patients with type 2 diabetes. Diabetes. 2005;**54**(3):603-608

[66] Cowin GJ, Jonsson JR, Bauer JD, et al. Magnetic resonance imaging and spectroscopy for monitoring liver steatosis. Journal of Magnetic Resonance Imaging. 2008;**28**(4):937-945

[67] Sjöström L, Lindroos AK, Peltonen M, et al. Lifestyle, diabetes, and cardiovascular risk factors 10 years after bariatric surgery. The New England Journal of Medicine. 2004;**351**(26):2683-2693

[68] Dixon JB, Bhathal PS, O'Brien PE. Weight loss and non-alcoholic fatty liver disease: Falls in gamma-glutamyl transferase concentrations are associated with histologic improvement. Obesity Surgery. 2006;**16**(10):1278-1286

[69] Silvestre V, Ruano M, Domínguez Y, et al. Morbid obesity and gastric bypass surgery: Biochemical profile. Obesity Surgery. 2004;**14**(9):1227-1232

[70] Stratopoulos C, Papakonstantinou A, Terzis I, et al. Changes in liver histology accompanying massive weight loss after gastroplasty for morbid obesity. Obesity Surgery. 2005;**15**(8):1154-1160

[71] Johansson HE, Haenni A, Ohrvall M, Sundbom M, Zethelius B. Alterations in proinsulin and insulin dynamics, HDL cholesterol and ALT after gastric bypass surgery. A 42-months follow-up study. Obesity Surgery. 2009;**19**(5):601-607

[72] Pontiroli AE, Pizzocri P, Librenti MC, et al. Laparoscopic adjustable gastric banding for the treatment of morbid (grade 3) obesity and its metabolic complications: A three-year study. The Journal of Clinical Endocrinology and Metabolism. 2002;**87**(8):3555-3561

[73] Burza MA, Romeo S, Kotronen A, et al. Long-term effect of bariatric surgery on liver enzymes in the Swedish obese subjects (SOS) study. PLoS One. 2013;**8**(3):e60495

[74] Hafeez S, Ahmed MH. Bariatric surgery as potential treatment for nonalcoholic fatty liver disease: A future treatment by choice or by chance? Journal of Obesity. 2013;**2013**:839275

[75] Mummadi RR, Kasturi KS, Chennareddygari S, Sood GK. Effect of bariatric surgery on nonalcoholic fatty liver disease: Systematic review and meta-analysis. Clinical Gastroenterology and Hepatology. 2008;**6**(12):1396-1402

[76] Estruch R, Ros E, Salas-Salvadó J, et al. Primary prevention of cardiovascular disease with a Mediterranean diet. The New England Journal of Medicine. 2013;**368**(14):1279-1290

[77] van Herpen NA, Schrauwen-Hinderling VB, Schaart G, Mensink RP, Schrauwen P. Three weeks on a high-fat diet increases intrahepatic lipid accumulation and decreases metabolic flexibility in healthy overweight men. The Journal of Clinical Endocrinology and Metabolism. 2011;**96**(4):E691-E695

[78] Gillingham LG, Harris-Janz S, Jones PJ. Dietary monounsaturated fatty acids are protective against metabolic syndrome and cardiovascular disease risk factors. Lipids. 2011;**46**(3):209-228

[79] Alonso A, Ruiz-Gutierrez V, Martínez-González MA. Monounsaturated fatty acids, olive oil and blood pressure: Epidemiological, clinical and experimental evidence. Public Health Nutrition. 2006;**9**(2):251-257

[80] Ryan MC, Itsiopoulos C, Thodis T, et al. The Mediterranean diet improves hepatic steatosis and insulin sensitivity in individuals with non-alcoholic fatty liver disease. Journal of Hepatology. 2013;**59**(1):138-143

[81] Bozzetto L, Prinster A, Annuzzi G, et al. Liver fat is reduced by an isoenergetic MUFA diet in a controlled randomized study in type 2 diabetic patients. Diabetes Care. 2012;**35**(7):1429-1435

[82] Mozaffarian D, Wu JH. Omega-3 fatty acids and cardiovascular disease: Effects on risk factors, molecular pathways, and clinical events. Journal of the American College of Cardiology. 2011;**58**(20):2047-2067

[83] Grimsgaard S, Bønaa KH, Hansen JB, Myhre ES. Effects of highly purified eicosapentaenoic acid and docosahexaenoic acid on hemodynamics in humans. The American Journal of Clinical Nutrition. 1998;**68**(1):52-59

[84] Bucher HC, Hengstler P, Schindler C, Meier G. N-3 polyunsaturated fatty acids in coronary heart disease: A meta-analysis of randomized controlled trials. The American Journal of Medicine. 2002;**112**(4):298-304

[85] Ooi EM, Lichtenstein AH, Millar JS, et al. Effects of therapeutic lifestyle change diets high and low in dietary fish-derived FAs on lipoprotein metabolism in middle-aged and elderly subjects. Journal of Lipid Research. 2012;**53**(9):1958-1967

[86] Bjermo H, Iggman D, Kullberg J, et al. Effects of n-6 PUFAs compared with SFAs on liver fat, lipoproteins, and inflammation in abdominal obesity: A randomized controlled trial. The American Journal of Clinical Nutrition. 2012;**95**(5):1003-1012

[87] Khaw KT, Friesen MD, Riboli E, Luben R, Wareham N. Plasma phospholipid fatty acid concentration and incident coronary heart disease in men and women: The EPIC-Norfolk prospective study. PLoS Medicine. 2012;**9**(7):e1001255

[88] Ooi EM, Ng TW, Watts GF, Barrett PH. Dietary fatty acids and lipoprotein metabolism: New insights and updates. Current Opinion in Lipidology. 2013;**24**(3):192-197

[89] McLaughlin T, Carter S, Lamendola C, et al. Effects of moderate variations in macronutrient composition on weight loss and reduction in cardiovascular disease risk in obese, insulin-resistant adults. The American Journal of Clinical Nutrition. 2006;**84**(4):813-821

[90] Foster GD, Wyatt HR, Hill JO, et al. A randomized trial of a low-carbohydrate diet for obesity. The New England Journal of Medicine. 2003;**348**(21):2082-2090

[91] Ryan MC, Abbasi F, Lamendola C, Carter S, McLaughlin TL. Serum alanine aminotransferase levels decrease further with carbohydrate than fat restriction in insulin-resistant adults. Diabetes Care. 2007;**30**(5):1075-1080

[92] Carter P, Khunti K, Davies MJ. Dietary recommendations for the prevention of type 2 diabetes: What are they based on? Journal of Nutrition and Metabolism. 2012;**2012**:847202

[93] Kim J, Tanabe K, Yokoyama N, Zempo H, Kuno S. Association between physical activity and metabolic syndrome in middle-aged Japanese: A cross-sectional study. BMC Public Health. 2011;**11**:624

[94] Johnson NA, George J. Fitness versus fatness: Moving beyond weight loss in nonalcoholic fatty liver disease. Hepatology. 2010;**52**(1):370-381

[95] Carroll JF, Franks SF, Smith AB, Phelps DR. Visceral adipose tissue loss and insulin resistance 6 months after laparoscopic gastric banding surgery: A preliminary study. Obesity Surgery. 2009;**19**(1):47-55

[96] Rector RS, Thyfault JP, Morris RT, et al. Daily exercise increases hepatic fatty acid oxidation and prevents steatosis in Otsuka long-Evans Tokushima fatty rats. American Journal of Physiology. Gastrointestinal and Liver Physiology. 2008;**294**(3):G619-G626

[97] Mikus CR, Rector RS, Arce-Esquivel AA, et al. Daily physical activity enhances reactivity to insulin in skeletal muscle arterioles of hyperphagic Otsuka long-Evans Tokushima fatty rats. Journal of Applied Physiology. 2010;**109**(4):1203-1210

[98] Shojaee-Moradie F, Baynes KC, Pentecost C, et al. Exercise training reduces fatty acid availability and improves the insulin sensitivity of glucose metabolism. Diabetologia. 2007;**50**(2):404-413

[99] Johnson NA, Sachinwalla T, Walton DW, et al. Aerobic exercise training reduces hepatic and visceral lipids in obese individuals without weight loss. Hepatology. 2009;**50**(4): 1105-1112

[100] van der Heijden GJ, Wang ZJ, Chu ZD, et al. A 12-week aerobic exercise program reduces hepatic fat accumulation and insulin resistance in obese, Hispanic adolescents. Obesity (Silver Spring). 2010;**18**(2):384-390

[101] Bonekamp S, Barone BB, Clark J, Stewart KJ. The effect of an exercise training intervention on hepatic steatosis. Hepatology. 2008;**48**(Suppl 1):806a

[102] Know your fats. American Heart Association website. http://www.heart.org/HEARTORG/Conditions/Cholesterol/PreventionTreatmentofHighCholesterol/Know-Your-Fats_UCM_305628_Article.jsp. [Accessed 06-06-2017]

[103] O'Donovan G, Kearney EM, Nevill AM, Woolf-May K, Bird SR. The effects of 24 weeks of moderate- or high-intensity exercise on insulin resistance. European Journal of Applied Physiology. 2005;**95**(5-6):522-528

[104] Kistler KD, Brunt EM, Clark JM, et al. Physical activity recommendations, exercise intensity, and histological severity of nonalcoholic fatty liver disease. The American Journal of Gastroenterology. 2011;**106**(3):460-468

[105] St George A, Bauman A, Johnston A, Farrell G, Chey T, George J. Independent effects of physical activity in patients with nonalcoholic fatty liver disease. Hepatology. 2009;**50**(1):68-76

[106] Chen SM, Liu CY, Li SR, Huang HT, Tsai CY, Jou HJ. Effects of therapeutic lifestyle program on ultrasound-diagnosed nonalcoholic fatty liver disease. Journal of the Chinese Medical Association. 2008;**71**(11):551-558

[107] de Mello MT, de Piano A, Carnier J, et al. Long-term effects of aerobic plus resistance training on the metabolic syndrome and adiponectinemia in obese adolescents. Journal of Clinical Hypertension (Greenwich, Conn.). 2011;**13**(5):343-350

[108] de Piano A, de Mello MT, Sanches LP, et al. Long-term effects of aerobic plus resistance training on the adipokines and neuropeptides in nonalcoholic fatty liver disease obese adolescents. European Journal of Gastroenterology and Hepatology. 2012;**24**(11):1313-1324

[109] Hallsworth K et al. Resistance exercise reduces liver fat and its mediators in non-alcoholic fatty liver disease independent of weight loss. Gut. DOI: 10.1136/gut.2011.242073

[110] Hasegawa T, Yoneda M, et al. Plasma transforming growth factor-beta1 level and efficacy of alpha-tocopherol in patients with non-alcoholic steatohepatitis: A pilot study. Alimentary Pharmacology & Therapeutics. 2001;**15**:1667-1672

[111] Kugelmas M, Hill DB, Vivian B, Marsano L, CJ MC. Cytokines and NASH : A pilot study of the effects of lifestyle modification and vitamin E. Hepatology. 2003;**38**:413-419

[112] Sanyal AJ, Chalasini N, Kowdley KV, et al. Pioglitazone, vitamin E, or placebo for nonalcoholic steatohepatitis. New England Journal of Medicine. 2010;**362**:16751685. DOI: 10.1056/NEJMoa0907929

[113] Arendt BM, Allard JP. Effect of atorvastatin, vitamin E and C on nonalcoholic fatty liver disease: is the combination required? The American Journal of Gastroenterology. 2011;**106**:78-80

[114] Sesso HD, Cook NR, Buring JE, Manson JE, Gaziano JM. Alcohol consumption and the risk of hypertension in women and men. Hypertension. 2008;**51**:1080-1087. DOI: 10.1161/HYPERTENSION AHA.107.104968

[115] Bjelakovic G, Nikolova D, Gluud LL, Simonetti RG, Gluud C. Antioxidant supplements for prevention of mortality in healthy participants and patients with various diseases. Cochrane Database of Systematic Reviews. 2012 Mar 14;**3**:CD007176. DOI: 10.1002/14651858.CD007176.pub2. Review

[116] Pittas AG, Harris SS, Stark PC, Dawson-Hughes B. The effects of calcium and vitamin D supplementation on blood glucose and markers of inflammation in non-diabetic adults. Diabetes Care. 2007;**30**:980-986

[117] Kendrick J, Targher G, Smits G, Chonchol M. 25-Hydroxyvitamin D deficiency is independently associated with cardiovascular disease in the third National Health and nutrition examination survey. Atherosclerosis. 2009;**205**:255-260

[118] Musso G, Anty R, Petta S. Antioxidant therapy and drugs interfering with lipid metabolism: could they be effective in NAFLD patients? Current Pharmaceutical Design. 2013;**19**:5297-5313

[119] Di Minno MN, Russolillo A, Lupoli R, Ambrosino P, Di Minno A, et al. Omega-3 fatty acids for the treatment of non-alcoholic fatty liver disease. World Journal of Gastroenterology. 2012;**18**:5839-5847

[120] Compare D, Coccoli P, Rocco A, Nardone OM, De Maria S, Cartenì M, et al. Gut–liver axis: The impact of gut microbiota on non-alcoholic fatty liver disease. Nutrition, Metabolism & Cardiovascular Diseases. 2012;**22**:471-476. DOI: 10.1016/j.numecd.2012.02.007

[121] Loguercio C, DeSimone T, Federico A, Terracciano F, Tuccillo C, DiChicco M, Carteni M. Gut-liver axis: A new point of attack to treat chronic liver damage? The American Journal of Gastroenterology. 2002;**97**:2144-2146

[122] Loguercio C, Federico A, Tuccillo C, Terracciano F, D'Auria MV, et al. Beneficial effects of a probiotic VSL#3 on parameters of liver dysfunction in chronic liver diseases. Journal of Clinical Gastroenterology. 2005;**39**:540-543

[123] Li X, Zhuo R, Tiong S, Di Cara F, King-Jones K, Hughes SC, Campbell SD, Wevrick R. The Smc5/Smc6/MAGE complex confers resistance to caffeine and genotoxic stress in Drosophila melanogaster. PLoS One. 2013;**8**(3):e59866

[124] Aller R, De Luis DA, Izaola O, Conde R, Gonzalez Sagrado M, Primo D, et al. Effect of a probiotic on liver aminotransferases in nonalcoholic fatty liver disease patients: A double blind randomized clinical trial. European Review for Medical and Pharmacological Sciences. 2011;**15**(9):1090e5

[125] Sahebkar A. Potential efficacy of ginger as a natural supplement for nonalcoholic fatty liver disease. World Journal of Gastroenterology. 2011 Jan 14;**17**(2):271-272. DOI: 10.3748/wjg.v17.i2.271

Chapter 8

Caffeine with Links to NAFLD and Accelerated Brain Aging

Ian James Martins

Additional information is available at the end of the chapter

http://dx.doi.org/10.5772/intechopen.70581

Abstract

Nutritional diets are essential to prevent nonalcoholic fatty liver disease (NAFLD) in the global obesity and diabetes epidemic. The ingestion of palmitic acid-rich diets induces NAFLD in animal and human studies. The beneficial properties of olive oil (oleic acid) may be superseded by ingestion of palmitic acid-rich diets. Hepatic caffeine metabolism is regulated by palmitic and oleic acid with effects of these fats on amyloid beta metabolism. Healthy fats such as olive oil may facilitate rapid amyloid beta clearance in the periphery to maintain drug therapy in diabetes and various neurological diseases. Repression of the anti-aging gene sirtuin 1 (Sirt 1) prevents the beneficial properties of olive oil. Brain disorders induce NAFLD and supersede caffeine's therapeutic effects in the prevention of NAFLD. Delayed hepatic caffeine metabolism in NAFLD and increased caffeine transport to the brain with aging-induced mitophagy in neurons with induction of type 3 diabetes and neurodegenerative disease.

Keywords: caffeine, nonalcoholic fatty liver disease, brain aging, palmitic acid, mitochondria

1. Introduction

The global increase in nonalcoholic fatty liver disease (NAFLD) is linked to various induction factors such as excessive caloric intake, genetic, environmental inducing factors and psychosocial factors that override the liver's ability to metabolize lipids and determine excess body fat (adipose tissue size) with the risk of dyslipidemia, obesity, cardiovascular disease, hypertension, and insulin resistance that lead to population mortality in developed countries. In developed countries, the Western diet is known to be high in fat and glucose and closely involved in early liver disease associated with excess transfer of fat to the adipose tissue (visceral fat) and the induction of the metabolic syndrome and obesity. Increased susceptibility to obesity in man compared with other species now indicates NAFLD to be the clinical condition involved in the induction of obesity in man [1–3]. In North America, the rate of childhood obesity has doubled in the last 20 years and similar statistics are reported in countries like Thailand, China, Brazil, and South Africa. The prevalence of childhood and adolescent obesity has increased since 1980 with concerns for NAFLD to exceed 50% of the childhood population [4–6]. Early dietary intervention in genetic and obese/diabetic mice models has indicated reversal and stabilization of NAFLD with relevance to the global NAFLD and neurodegeneration. Education programs such as food restriction programs (**Figure 1**) have been performed but induction of global NAFLD has not decreased in the world [7, 8]. The projected health care costs by the year 2018 in relation to obesity/diabetes-related medical expenses in the United States have been reported to be 344 billion dollars accounting for 21% of total health care costs. Excessive caloric intake, genetic, environmental inducing agents, and psychosocial factors all contribute to the cause of NAFLD (**Figure 1**) with the reduced metabolism of lipids involved in the development of obesity in middle adult life. In the global population, the prevalence of NAFLD has increased from 15% in 1980 to 25% in 2010 with NAFLD to increase to 40% of the global population by the year 2050. In the developing world, the increased obesity/diabetes epidemic is now associated with diet and the presence of specific chemicals such as xenobiotics [9]. The interactions between the brain, liver, and adipose tissue are defective [10] with reduced adipose tissue-liver crosstalk [10–12] responsible for the defective hepatic metabolism of dietary fat, xenobiotics, and drugs and related to the induction of global NAFLD epidemic. Major interests in caffeine intake have accelerated with relevance to global mitophagy, amyloid beta aggregation, NAFLD, and neurodegenerative

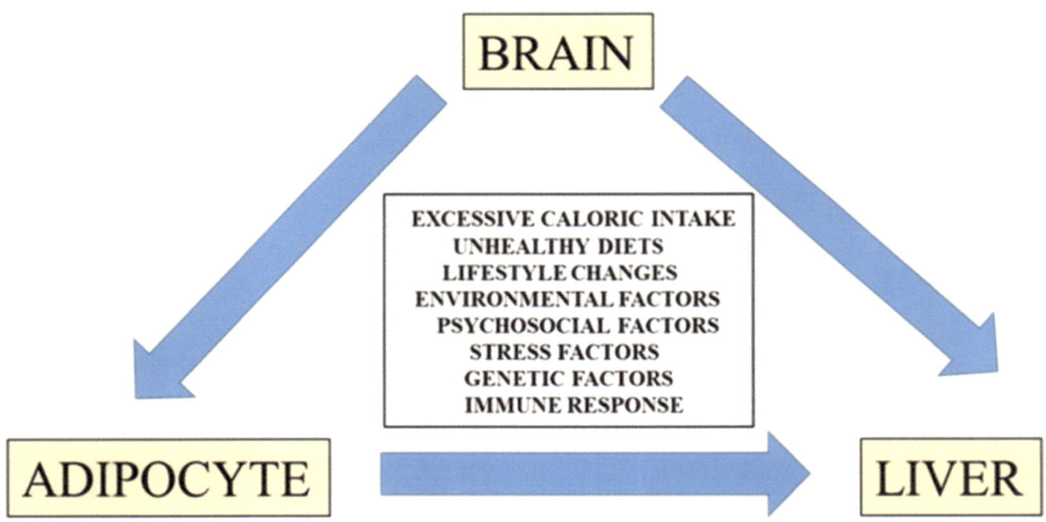

Figure 1. Inducing factors for NAFLD override the brain regulation of the adipose tissue-liver crosstalk. The dose of caffeine used in healthy diets has become important with relevance to the brain control of liver function. Palmitic acid-rich diets induce NAFLD and delay caffeine metabolism with increased caffeine transport to the brain. Other factors such as stress and psychosocial factors disturb brain function with altered cellular lipid metabolism which is now linked to obesity and the NAFLD epidemic.

http://dx.doi.org/10.5772/intechopen.70581

disease [13]. Caffeine is an appetite suppressant with effects on improving liver fat metabolism and adipogenesis [14] and important to the adipose tissue-liver crosstalk. Brain regulation of the adipose tissue-liver crosstalk is impaired by various inducing factors with excess transport of caffeine to the brain that interferes with the circadian rhythm with relevance to accelerated aging [14–17]. Inducing factors for NAFLD (**Figure 1**) override the beneficial effects of caffeine on adipocyte/liver fat metabolism [18, 19] and the dose of caffeine used in diets has become important with relevance to the NAFLD epidemic since the pharmacokinetics of caffeine may be completely impaired in the liver (NAFLD) in overweight/obese individuals [2, 20–27].

Unhealthy diets (**Figure 1**) that contain palmitic acid (cream, butter, and cheese) increase cholesterol levels and induce NAFLD [28–32] and neurodegeneration with complete impairment of caffeine actions with relevance to its role as a modulator of receptors relevant to the adipose tissue and liver fat metabolism. Palmitic acid diets alter cell cholesterol and phospholipid dynamics with increased contents of phospholipids such as dipalmitoylphosphatidylcholine (DPPC) that are relevant to increased membrane cholesterol content [33, 34] with relevance to delayed hepatic caffeine and amyloid beta transport and metabolism. Palmitic acid and DPPC have major effects on membrane cholesterol formation that stimulate amyloid beta formation [35, 36]. Amyloid beta is a 4-kDa hydrophobic peptide (**Figure 2**) released from neurons in the brain for metabolism by the liver [37] with recent research that caffeine (hydrophobic

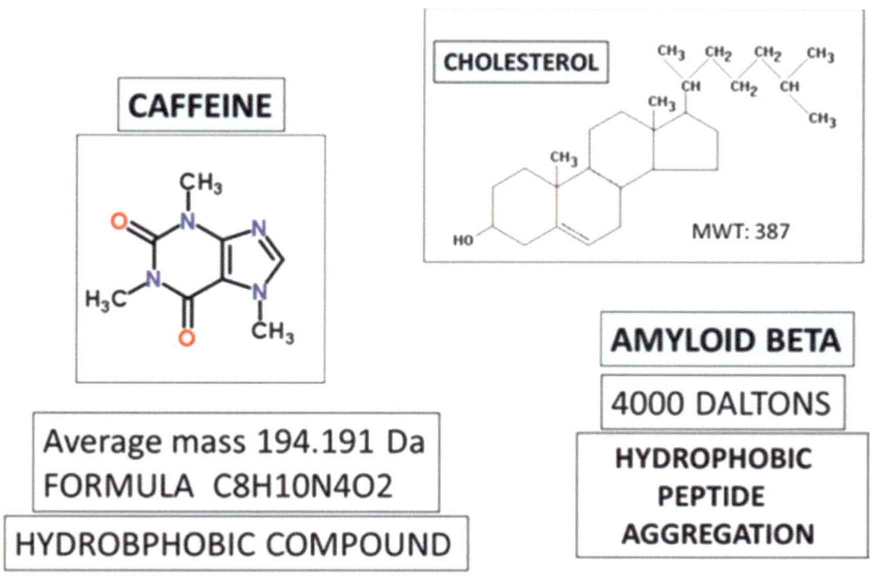

Figure 2. Increased cholesterol levels have been associated with toxic amyloid beta formation. Diets with increased palmitic acid increase cell cholesterol and the phospholipid dipalmitoylphosphatidylcholine (DPPC) with relevance to delayed cell amyloid beta transport and caffeine metabolism. Caffeine is a hydrophobic compound and its increased insertion into the cell membrane with aging is related to abnormal cholesterol and amyloid beta metabolism with the induction of mitophagy. The consumption of olive oil (oleic acid) is associated with the phospholipid 1-palmitoyl-2-oleolylphosphatidylcholine (POPC) and is related to rapid amyloid beta and caffeine metabolism.

compound, **Figure 2**) improves brain-liver amyloid beta transport and metabolism with the prevention of neurodegeneration [38, 39]. DPPC/cholesterol interactions accumulate cellular caffeine with corruption of the brain-liver amyloid beta metabolism with accelerated brain aging associated with toxic amyloid beta aggregation (**Figure 2**). Increased cell phospholipid dynamics with consumption of olive oil (oleic acid) are associated with phospholipids such as 1-palmitoyl-2-oleolylphosphatidylcholine (POPC) that is a common pattern of naturally occurring phospholipids in cells and relevant to cell phospholipid dynamics [40] and rapid caffeine metabolism. Palmitic acid and DPPC are sensitive to cholesterol with toxic effects involved in the interference with brain-liver amyloid beta and caffeine metabolism with relevance to caffeine-induced mitophagy [41, 42] and the induction of NAFLD and neurodegeneration in global communities.

2. Defective adipose tissue-liver crosstalk in the induction of the global NAFLD epidemic

New quantitative genetic methods such as the use of DNA and RNA microarrays have been used to examine novel genetic pathways and now identify a single gene to be involved in the NAFLD and obesity epidemic. The anti-aging gene sirtuin 1 (Sirt 1) has now been implicated as a NAD(+)-dependent class III histone deacetylase (HDAC) protein that targets transcription factors to adapt gene expression to metabolic activity, insulin resistance, and inflammation in chronic diseases [43–46]. Sirt 1 is involved in food intake regulation [47, 48], gluconeogenesis in the liver [49], fat mobilization from white adipose tissue, cholesterol metabolism, and energy metabolism [50, 51]. In adipose tissue, Sirt 1 activates fat mobilization by inhibiting peroxisome proliferator-activated receptor gamma (PPAR-gamma) [52, 53] and in the pancreas Sirt 1 repression decreases insulin secretion with effects on beta cell uncoupling protein 2 levels [54]. Sirt 1 influences mitochondrial biogenesis in the adipose tissue and liver with relevance to NAFLD [10]. Furthermore, diet and nutrigenomics are involved in Sirt 1 regulation of DNA repair with transcription factors regulated by Sirt 1 connected to the nuclear receptors such as peroxisome proliferator-activated receptor (PPARalpha, PPARgamma), liver X receptor, pregnane X receptor, and farnesoid X receptor involved in liver metabolic homeostasis with roles in lipid metabolism in adipose tissue [9].

The effects of dysregulated Sirt 1 on adipocyte differentiation [55–59] and regulation of gene expression involves the secretion of adiponectin [60–62] with adipocyte size negatively correlated with adiponectin levels, adipose tissue ceramide metabolism, and HDL levels [63–67]. Adiponectin is mainly secreted from the adipose tissue into the bloodstream and inversely correlated with body fat in adults. Adiponectin self-associates into larger structures from trimers to form hexamers or dodecamers with the high-molecular weight form, biologically more active with regard to glucose homeostasis. High fat intake is associated with decreased adiponectin levels [68] and downregulation of Sirt 1 [10] with low adiponectin levels associated with the metabolic syndrome, NAFLD [69–71] with effects on hypercholesterolemia (low high-density lipoproteins, apolipoprotein AI levels and high low-density lipoprotein, apolipoprotein B levels) associated with insulin resistance and NAFLD (**Figure 3**). Adiponectin

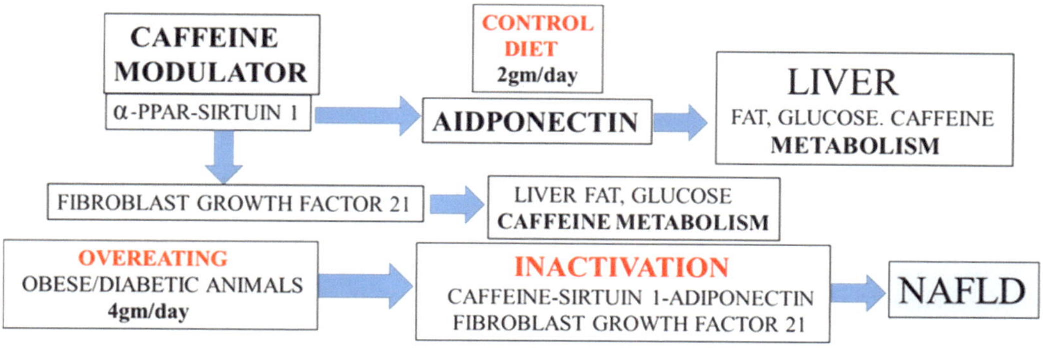

Figure 3. Dietary fat consumption in man needs to be carefully controlled to allow caffeine to modulate cell Sirtuin 1 activity that is involved in mitochondrial biogenesis and the metabolism of cellular fatty acids. Diets that are low in calories activate Sirtuin 1 and allow caffeine-induced modulation of adiponectin levels essential for the adipose tissue-liver crosstalk and the hepatic metabolism of glucose and fatty acids. In rodents, feeding mice 2 g/day instead of 4 g/day increases hepatic fatty acid metabolism and activates hepatic Sirtuin 1 involved in glucose and fatty acid metabolism. Sirtuin 1 is involved in adipose tissue-liver FGF21 production essential for mitochondrial function in the brain and the metabolism of fatty acids, glucose, and caffeine in the liver. The calculated fat content by (Martins IJ, author) in man is related to between 20 and 30 g/day and fat intake at this consumption rate is essential for the prevention of NAFLD.

deficiency has been shown to reduce hepatic ATP-binding cassette transporter ABCA1 (ABCA1) and apo AI synthesis with relevance to the reverse cholesterol transport [72]. FGF21 is now associated with NAFLD [73–76] with hepatic FGF21 shown to regulate lipolysis (fatty acid release) with FGF21 critical in the reduction of adipose tissue ceramides. In insulin resistance and AD, FGF21 and adiponectin levels are implicated in increased cellular ceramide levels and NAFLD [77–81] associated with cholesterol displacement in membranes [82–84] with relevance to amyloid beta aggregation [85]. Sirt 1/adiponectin/FGF21 dysregulation determine hepatic cholesterol metabolism with effects on plasma apo B levels mediated via Sirt 1 and transcription factor C/EBPalpha, which regulates the transcription of the apo B gene [85]. Adipocytes from obese and diabetic individuals are associated with increased adipocyte APP gene expression and plasma amyloid beta levels that implicate adiponectin and Sirt 1 dysregulation with cholesterol and amyloid beta metabolism [86–90]. High-calorie diets downregulate Sirt 1 with reduced adiponectin expression in obesity and diabetes [91] associated with adipose tissue transformation and liver development [60, 86]. Fasting and feeding regulate PPAR alpha-Sirt 1 expression related to hepatic FGF21 production and have become important to NAFLD and the metabolic syndrome [85]. FGF21 is an important activator of Sirt 1-mediated release of adiponectin [85]. FGF21 binds to FGF receptor and beta klotho receptor complex [85] and activates adipose tissue Sirt 1 by increase in NAD+ and activation of peroxisome proliferator-activated receptor gamma coactivator 1-alpha (PGC1-alpha) and AMP-activated protein kinase (AMPK). Unhealthy diets and Sirt 1 repression effect the release of adipose tissue adipokines (adiponectin and leptin) and cytokines (tumor necrosis factor alpha, interleukin-6 and C-reactive protein levels, and Ang II) [92] with FGF21 [73–76] implicated in NAFLD and other chronic diseases associated with accelerated brain aging. In man, caffeine has been associated with increased adiponectin levels with relevance to beneficial effects on liver function [93, 94]. Caffeine and its effects on the adipose tissue-liver crosstalk involve caffeine related to adipose tissue adiponectin release essential for liver function. Caffeine is a modulator of histone deacetylase and its effects as a histone deacetylase modulator [27, 95] in the adipose tissue-liver crosstalk involve the dose of caffeine that is of critical importance to Sirt 1/adiponectin release [85, 96, 97] essential to maintain hepatic metabolism of fatty acids and glucose [18, 98]. Caffeine is important to reduce inflammatory processes [99, 100] with adipose tissue transformation and release of inflammatory cytokines that induce NAFLD [100]. Sirt 1 is involved in autoimmunity [101, 102] with relevance to regulation of various immune cell events in the adipose tissue and liver.

Assessment of hepatic lipid metabolism has been extensively conducted in obese and diabetic rodents with relevance to NAFLD in man [103–107]. In rodents with diets (5% fat), the intake of food per day was approximately 2 g/day and the hepatic metabolism of injected labeled lipoproteins was rapid and cleared and metabolized from the blood plasma within 30 min. In obese and diabetic rodents that had appetite dysregulation consumed approximately 4 g/day (**Figure 3**), the hepatic clearance and metabolism of fats were defective. The excess and ingested fat in obese/diabetic rodents completely downregulated hepatic Sirt 1 with relevance to the NAFLD that develops in these mice with the aging process. In Sirt 1 knockout mice [108, 109], NAFLD develops with relevance to the importance of Sirt 1 in liver fat and cholesterol metabolism [110]. The primary role of fat intake was assessed in obese/diabetic mice that were only allowed to consume 2 g/day (**Figure 3**) instead of 4 g/day and hepatic lipid metabolism was improved in these obese/diabetic rodent experiments with relevance to calorie-sensitive regulation of hepatic Sirt 1 (**Figure 3**). Dietary fat consumption in man needs to be carefully controlled to allow caffeine/adiponectin effects to prevent the induction of NAFLD. The calculated fat content in man has now been determined by author's calculations to be approximately 20–30 g/day [13] and differs from other international researchers [111]. In several laboratories, cellular cholesterol levels are associated with increased amyloid beta formation in the brain and periphery [37], and Sirt 1 downregulation is associated with defective caffeine and cholesterol metabolism (**Figure 4**) with relevance to hepatic amyloid beta clearance and induction of NAFLD [112]. Increased plasma caffeine levels displace amyloid beta and fatty acids from albumin by competition for albumin binding sites [113] with relevance to amyloid beta aggregation [114]. Increased caffeine membrane levels in the liver and brain may affect cholesterol efflux with toxic amyloid beta aggregation (**Figure 4**) relevant to cell apoptosis. Sirt 1 is essential for neuron proliferation with effects of excess cell caffeine that interferes with cell magnesium levels (**Figure 4**) and supersedes the anti-amyloid beta aggregation properties of caffeine [115]. Magnesium deficiency has been associated with hypercholesterolemia and induction of NAFLD [116]. Magnesium is now relevant to maintenance of peripheral hepatic amyloid beta metabolism with magnesium levels critical to the prevention of high-cell cholesterol-induced amyloid beta formation. In NAFLD (**Figure 4**), caffeine consumption should be carefully controlled to prevent magnesium deficiency [117] and to assist with the reduction in hepatic fibrosis in NAFLD [118].

Palmitic acid-rich diets (20–30 g fat/day) should carefully calculate palmitic acid consumption per day to prevent interference of the adipose tissue-crosstalk and induction of NAFLD [13]. Palmitic acid is an Sirt 1 inhibitor [119, 120] with induction of cell cholesterol efflux disturbances

http://dx.doi.org/10.5772/intechopen.70581

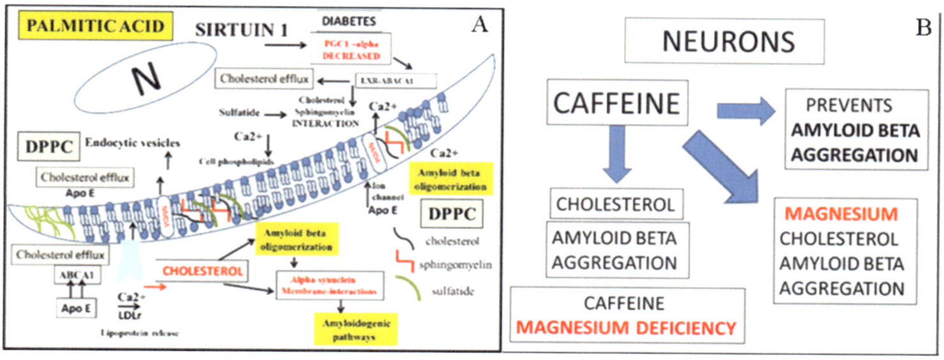

Figure 4. In panel A, palmitic acid as an inhibitor of Sirt 1 is associated with defective caffeine and cholesterol metabolism with relevance to hepatic amyloid beta clearance and induction of NAFLD. Cell caffeine levels are associated with calcium-induced amyloid beta oligomer formation with mitophagy in the liver and brain. In panel B, irreversible effects with aging of palmitic acid induce cell DPPC/cholesterol formation and interfere with caffeine's anti-amyloid beta oligomer properties with increased cell caffeine levels related to magnesium deficiency (NAFLD) and increased cholesterol associated amyloid beta aggregation.

relevant to cell amyloid beta-induced mitophagy [121] with liver inflammation. Palmitic acid induces DPPC phospholipid/cholesterol membrane changes that delay caffeine metabolism with increased cell caffeine levels associated with calcium-induced amyloid beta oligomer formation in the liver and brain [27]. Palmitic acid converts to glucose in cells and with increased palmitic acid levels that are not controlled with aging may inactivate cell Sirt 1 glucose regulation (gluconeogenesis) and nullify the brain to liver amyloid beta clearance pathway with defective adipose tissue-liver crosstalk [10] relevant to induction of chronic diseases.

The gene-environment interaction identifies Sirt 1 in many global populations as the defective gene involved in the defective nuclear-mitochondria interactions in the adipose tissue and the liver relevant to the mitochondrial theory of aging [10]. Sirt 1 targets transcription factors such as peroxisome proliferator-activated receptor gamma coactivator 1-alpha (PGC1-alpha) and p53 to adapt gene expression to mitochondrial function by deacetylation of PGC1-alpha and p53 transcription factors [10], which are important to mitochondrial DNA homeostasis and mitochondrial biogenesis [122–126]. Inhibitors and activators of Sirt 1 [112] have been identified that may override caffeine and its role as a Sirt 1 modulator [27, 95, 112]. Inhibitors include alcohol, sirtinol, suramin and activators include leucine, pyruvic acid, and alpha-lipoic acid. These inhibitors may induce mitochondrial apoptosis and may override the adipose tissue-liver interaction with the induction of NAFLD. Sirt 1 is now referred to as the heat-shock gene with its critical role in heat-shock protein (HSP) metabolism [127, 128]. HSP is a chaperone for amyloid beta and with Sirt 1 repression is important to HSP-amyloid beta-induced endoplasmic reticulum stress relevant to mitophagy and induction of NAFLD [129, 130]. *Caenorhabditis elegans* sirtuins have similar homology to human Sirt 1 with relevance to effects of caffeine on Sirt 1 circadian dysregulation [129]. Induction of HSP from cells in the nematode *C. elegans* has been used for toxicological studies and indicates caffeine doses that induce HSP release with relevance to programmed cell death [129].

3. Accelerated brain aging and type 3 diabetes-induced NAFLD and chronic diseases

In the developed and developing world, the induction of NAFLD has become one of the major interests with its primary or secondary role in the induction of various chronic diseases. Accelerated brain aging with appetite dysregulation indicates that NAFLD may play a secondary role in the induction of various chronic diseases (**Figure 5**). Mitophagy and the induction of neurodegeneration with ****type 3 diabetes are now the primary defects with accelerated NAFLD connected to various chronic diseases (**Figure 5**). Major concerns for suprachiasmatic nucleus (SCN) defects in the hypothalamus may involve appetite dysregulation [11], core-body temperature defects [131], and whole-body glucose disorders (type 3 diabetes) may induce toxicity to the liver and various other organs. Factors such as stress, psychosocial, environmental factors [9], and sleep disorders [132] disturb SCN regulation of the circadian rhythm with toxic effects of glucose, cholesterol, caffeine, and amyloid beta levels to the brain and various tissues (**Figure 5**). Higher brain dysregulation corrupts the hypothalamus-pituitary axis, sympathetic and nonsympathetic pathways that have direct neural innervation to organs such as the liver. Defective hepatic caffeine metabolism may induce magnesium deficiency, apelinergic system imbalances [133, 134], interference with sympathetic pathways [26] connected to mitophagy, and various chronic diseases.

The ingestion of the amount of fat is critical to the adipose tissue-liver cross with immune reactivity [10, 135] connected to mitophagy and induction of NAFLD. Multiple theories of aging have been proposed and the immune theory of aging may involve adipose tissue transformation with activation of immune responses that involve macrophages and immune cells that lead to liver inflammation [10, 99] and the induction of NAFLD. The defect in the neural loop (autonomic nervous system) between the brain and adipose tissue [136] now may be

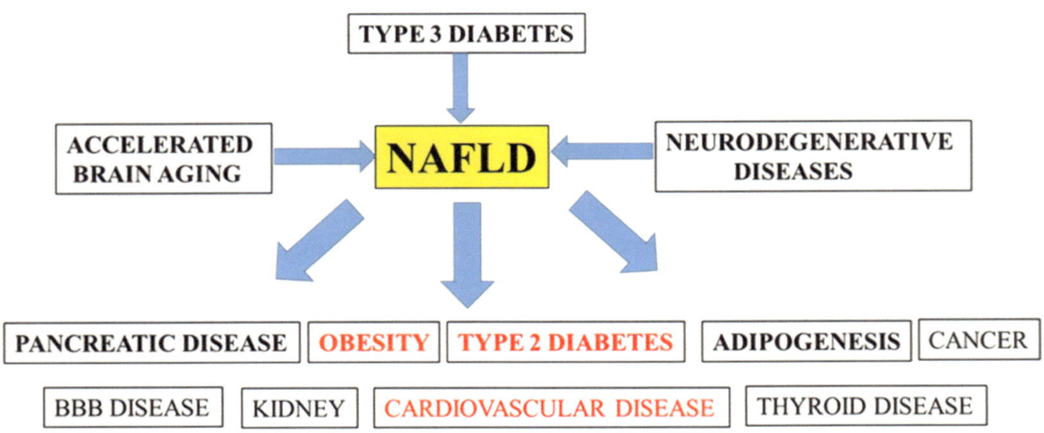

Figure 5. Defects in the suprachiasmatic nucleus (SCN) that involve appetite dysregulation, core-body temperature defects, and whole-body glucose disorders (type 3 diabetes) may induce NAFLD and various other chronic diseases. The primary role in the induction of NAFLD may be related to mitophagy-induced neurodegeneration with relevance to circadian rhythm disorders and complete nullification of hepatic caffeine metabolism by interference with the adipose tissue-liver crosstalk.

related to immunometabolism disorders with adipose tissue transformation. The nature of dietary fat with relevance to adipose tissue as the organ most susceptible to programmed cell death pathways involves transformation that is now important to determine the release of adipocyte inflammatory cytokines, hormones, and heat-shock proteins (HSP) that trigger liver inflammation and NAFLD in global communities [135]. Immunometabolism and accelerated aging are now connected to the adipose tissue and liver crosstalk with the mitochondria theory of aging important to both immune function [10] and metabolism of fats in the adipose tissue and liver. The transcription factor p53 is involved in immune responses, metabolism, and mitochondrial apoptosis [10, 123, 125] with diet, drugs, and environment [9] critical to the regulation of Sirt 1/p53 immunometabolism and induction of NAFLD in the developed world.

Rapid urbanization from 20 to 60% has occurred in Africa, India, China, and Asia and possibly involved with the large global diabetic population in these developing countries. The number of people with diabetes is projected to be double in Africa, Asia, and India. In Asia, the diabetic epidemic has escalated and accounts for 60% of the world diabetic population [137]. The diabetic epidemic has been associated with NAFLD in developing countries of Latin America, Asia [138], India, and Africa with prevalence (20–40%) [9] similar to developed countries [138–141]. Evidence from various studies [9] indicates that environmental factors (xenobiotics) are the major determinants of the increasing rate of diabetes (**Figure 6**). Major threats of xenobiotics such as environmental pollutants may increase with age in individuals

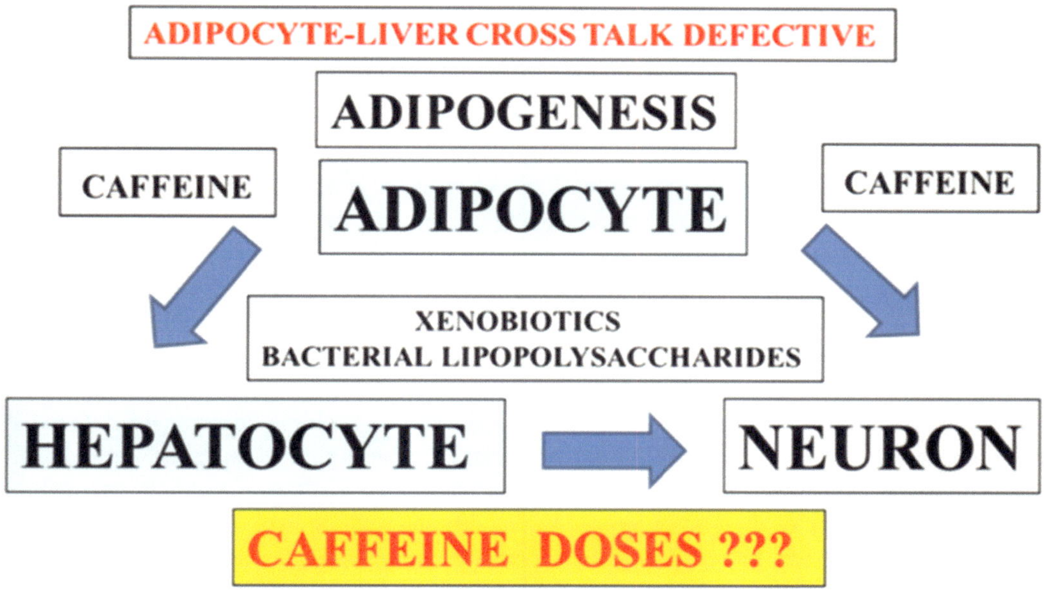

Figure 6. Caffeine is essential for the release of adiponectin from adipose tissue in obesity but the therapeutic effects of caffeine may be superseded with relevance to adipogenesis disorders. In the developing world, xenobiotics induce mitophagy in the adipose tissue and liver and supersede caffeine's protective effects on the mitochondria. In the developing world, plasma LPS levels have increased with effects on the induction of NAFLD and interference with neuron function. Caffeine doses should be carefully controlled with relevance to LPS cell membrane transformations that override caffeine and cell membrane interactions and promote caffeine effects on albumin involved in amyloid beta and fatty acid transport between the brain and the liver.

from developing countries. The NAFLD epidemic is connected to unhealthy diets and reduced hepatic xenobiotic metabolism with blood-brain barrier disorders [9] involved with interference of brain Sirt 1's role in DNA repair [10] with the induction of neuronal apoptosis and type 3 diabetes. The association between xenobiotics in food and the beneficial effects of caffeine (Sirt 1 modulation) on insulin resistance [142, 143] may be superseded with caffeine consumption in these individuals to be revised with relevance to toxic xenobiotic effects associated with delayed caffeine metabolism relevant to NAFLD and neurodegenerative diseases.

The interests in bacterial lipopolysaccharides (LPS) and their influence on cell membrane fluidity in the brain has accelerated with the increase in plasma LPS levels in individuals (30%) of the developing world [144, 145]. LPS is a critical repressor of Sirt 1 actions with the induction of dyslipidemia, mitophagy, and NAFLD [145]. LPS from Gram-negative bacteria is an amphiphile (covalently linked segments, surface carbohydrate polymer O-specific chain, core oligosaccharide, Lipid A) that can rapidly insert into cell membranes and transform mammalian cells. LPS may supersede POPC properties of the cell membrane and induce amyloid beta oligomerization [144].

4. Nutritional diets maintain brain and adipose tissue-liver crosstalk with prevention of NAFLD

In developed world, the consumption of fat consumed in man is between 44 and 78 g/day [111, 146]. The amount of fat consumed (20–30 g/day) is critical to maintain the brain regulation of the adipose tissue-liver crosstalk and connected to the maintenance of the circadian rhythm (12 h light/12 h dark cycle) that is critical to hepatic amyloid beta and glucose metabolism [147, 148]. The SCN is controlled by Sirt 1 with its dysfunction connected to brain circuitry disorders (**Figure** 7) and disconnections between the autonomic nervous system and the liver [148]. The amount of fat consumed with the aging process inactivates the effects of caffeine by interfering with hepatic caffeine metabolism with increased transport to the brain (**Figure 7**). In the brain, SCN neurons are sensitive to caffeine [149] with complete inactivation of the brain to adipose tissue-liver crosstalk and interfere with caffeine's beneficial effects on the sympathetic nervous system and reversal of NAFLD. Caffeine and its role in thermogenesis by modulation of mitochondrial function versus mitochondrial apoptosis are relevant to the consumption of various fats and diets in the developed and developing world. Sirt 1 is now referred as the gene involved in mitochondrial biogenesis that is critical to maintain cell function with the prevention of cell apoptosis [9–12, 122–125]. Sirt 1 is critical to SCN function and the maintenance of core-body temperature with essential control of the adipose tissue-liver crosstalk [131, 150]. The consumption of coconut oil (saturated fat) and palm oil (palmitic acid) should be carefully evaluated in individuals with core-body temperature disorders. These fats are solid at temperatures between 20 and 24°C and with abnormal body temperature dysregulation may be involved in the induction of NAFLD when compared with the consumption of olive oil (monounsaturated) that is liquid at a temperature (4°C) [130, 150]. Fish contains high levels of omega-3 fatty acids, docosahexaenoic acid (DHA 22:6n-3), and eicosapentaenoic acid (EPA 20:5n-3). These fatty acids are essential for liver fat metabolism with prevention of NAFLD [151, 152] and brain function but with changes in core body temperature (**Figure 7**), therapeutic lipids essential for the prevention of NAFLD may be completely inactivated [130, 131, 150]. Palmitic acid content in milk should be carefully controlled to allow the therapeutic effects of caffeine with relevance to mitochondrial thermogenesis and SCN regulation (**Figure 7**). Nutritional diets with timed meals are important for the prevention of NAFLD and with consumption of essential foods which include protein, eggs, cottage cheese, dairy, red meat, poultry, legumes, nuts, and seeds. These foods may contain minerals such as magnesium and zinc that are needed by many enzymes involved with DNA replication and repair with total magnesium intake that should be between 400 mg and 800 mg/day. Zinc deficiency has been reported in global communities with both minerals important to prevent liver and brain diseases and to allow effective vitamin and caffeine therapy. Vitamins such as vitamin B12, folic acid, vitamin B6, vitamins C, D, and E are essential to maintain liver and brain function. The consumption of phosphatidylinositol (PI) (g/day) is essential and lack of PI may not allow the maintenance of SCN function and whole body glucose homeostasis. In individuals with strenuous exercise, the PI half-life is rapid and may require PI ingestion of (g/day) to prevent amyloid beta aggregation and induction of NAFLD [153, 154]. Strenuous exercise may induce magnesium deficiency [116] and magnesium consumption needs revision to prevent SCN disturbances with type 3 diabetes and NAFLD.

The major defects with relevance to the global NAFLD epidemic involve the defective brain circadian circuitry and the adipose tissue-liver crosstalk [136, 155]. The SCN control of the

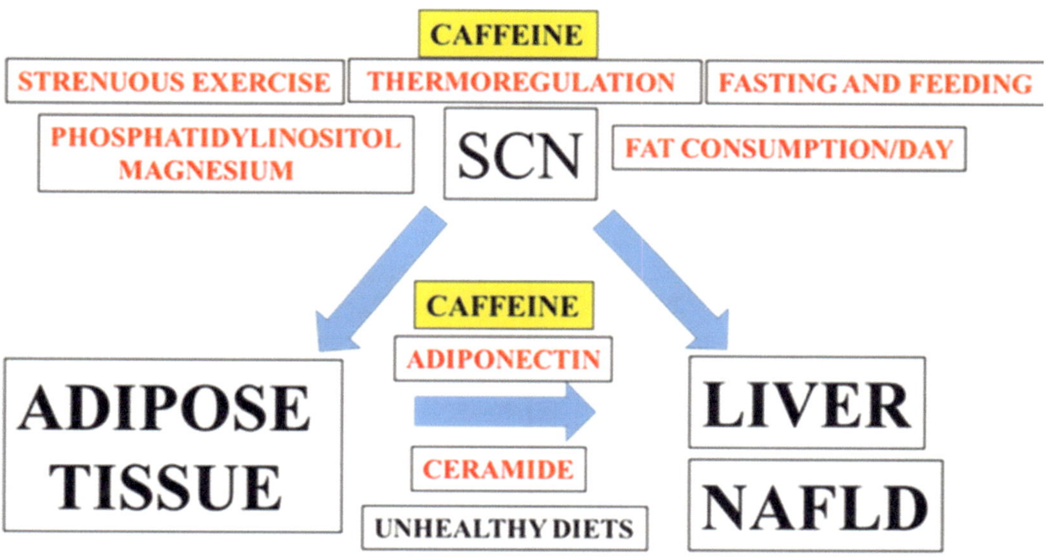

Figure 7. In the current global NAFLD epidemic, plasma ceramides indicate that the adipose tissue-liver crosstalk is completely defective with the release of toxic ceramides into the blood plasma. Sirt 1 downregulation is possibly connected to cell ceramide formation with adipose tissue disorders, liver steatosis development, and complete inactivation of caffeine's involvement in the prevention of NAFLD [94]. Integration of factors such as stress, sleep disorders, and environmental factors (strenuous exercise) inactivate the SCN regulation of the circadian rhythm with toxic effects of glucose, cholesterol, caffeine, and amyloid beta levels to mitochondria in various peripheral tissues.

adipose tissue metabolism allows adipocyte adiponectin release with essential effects on liver glucose and lipid homeostasis [155]. Sirt 1 and its modulation by caffeine have become important with caffeine involved in increased adiponectin levels in man. Apart from caffeine, other foods have been assessed to increase adiponectin levels such as omega-3 supplementation, fruit intake, green tea, magnesium, and hypolipidemic drugs are all involved in the modification of adiponectin levels [156–159]. In individuals with NAFLD, long-term dietary salt restriction is essential to increase adiponectin levels. Fasting and feeding is essential to maintain SCN circadian regulation of liver function that involves peripheral glucose homeostasis with adiponectin release critical to maintain insulin sensitivity and prevent NAFLD [85]. Gamma PPAR-Sirt 1 function in adipocytes is critical to adiponectin release with low adiponectin levels unsuitable to the maintenance of liver ceramide levels that are toxic to the liver and involved in insulin resistance. Ceramide levels and NAFLD [81–84] are now closely linked with programmed cell death. Alcohol consumption should be carefully controlled (Sirt 1 inhibition) with relevance to adiponectin levels in man [160]. Pyruvic acid, leucine, quercetin, green tea catechins, grape seed extract, curcumin, alpha lipoic acid, and resveratrol are Sirt 1 activators essential for SCN maintenance and the adipose tissue-liver cross talk. High-protein diets should be avoided to reduce amyloid beta formation by cells and to reduce the arginine content of the diet that switches leucine (Sirt 1 activator) for arginine in cells and tissues [132].

High-fiber diets [37] in various foods have become important with the consumption of phytosterols [37] involved in reducing intestinal cholesterol absorption and increased hepatic cholesterol metabolism relevant to the prevention of NAFLD in man. Phytosterols should be consumed (1–2 g/day) and excessive intake of phytosterols leads to neurotoxicity with neurodegeneration [37]. Phytosterols cross the blood–brain barrier in neurons to maintain neuron amyloid beta homeostasis [161]. Consumption of plant-based foods essential for phytosterol ingestion should be assessed for caffeine content since approximately 40 caffeine containing plants have been reported. Other caffeine containing foods such as coca cola, energy drinks, caffeine tablets, dark chocolate, chocolate chips, and energy mints should be assessed for caffeine content (mg). Vegetarians should carefully regulate phytosterol consumption over their lifespan to prevent interference with the beneficial effects of caffeine on cholesterol metabolism with relevance to NAFLD [37]. Excessive fructose consumption (fruit, fruit juices) should be avoided with fructose reported as a Sirt 1 inhibitor [162, 163] with the induction of NAFLD. In the developing world, very low carbohydrate diets should be consumed to prevent the absorption of LPS into the blood stream with beneficial effects on magnesium deficiency and the induction of NAFLD [164]. Diets with low-fat contents and without alcohol are essential to prevent the transport of LPS into lipoproteins and proteins in the blood plasma. LPS interferes with the SCN and adipose tissue-liver crosstalk [10, 85, 135, 136] and delays hepatic drug metabolism [165, 166] with premature brain aging and chronic disease progression (**Figure 6**). LPS induces changes in plasma albumin contents [112] in individuals in the developing world with relevance to interference with caffeine and its therapeutic properties with relevance to SCN regulation of adipose tissue-liver crosstalk. In recent studies, caffeine intake and glucose dyshomeostasis that supersede insulin therapy [142, 143] has raised concerns with relevance to glucose/amyloid beta-induced mitochondrial apoptosis and the induction of NAFLD. In the global chronic disease, adiponectin levels are low and to prevent mitochondrial apoptosis, a number of agents are required to maintain mitochondrial function and to prevent cell apoptosis. Diets that contain magnesium, pyrroloquinoline, quinone, resveratrol, and rutin stimulate mitochondrial biogenesis essential to stimulate SCN neuron mitochondrial function [167] with relevance to the global NAFLD epidemic and chronic diseases.

5. Conclusion

In global world, diabetes and mitochondrial disease are expected to cost the developing world US $400 million in the next 30 years. The quality of food consumed has raised major concerns with mitochondrial apoptosis linked to programmed cell death and nonalcoholic fatty liver disease (NAFLD). The amount, nature, and time of day of fat consumption are essential to maintain mitochondrial biogenesis. In the developed and developing world, nutritional interventions are essential to prevent NAFLD and ingestion of caffeine (appetite suppressant) that is associated with the prevention of adipocyte dysfunction and linked to liver function may be completely inactivated by unhealthy diets. In the developing world, bacterial lipopolysaccharides (LPS) may override healthy fat consumption and induce NAFLD. In the developing world, diets that contain LPS, mycotoxins, and xenobiotics interfere with caffeine metabolism with relevance to mitophagy and induction of NAFLD relevant to the survival of various species and man.

Acknowledgements

This work was supported by grants from Edith Cowan University, the McCusker Alzheimer's Research Foundation, and the National Health and Medical Research Council.

Author details

Ian James Martins[1,2,3]

Address all correspondence to: i.martins@ecu.edu.au

1 Centre of Excellence in Alzheimer's Disease Research and Care, School of Medical and Health Sciences, Edith Cowan University, Joondalup, Australia

2 School of Psychiatry and Clinical Neurosciences, The University of Western Australia, Nedlands, Australia

3 McCusker Alzheimer's Research Foundation, Hollywood Medical Centre, Nedlands, Australia

References

[1] de la Monte SM, Longato L, Tong M, Wands JR. Insulin resistance and neurodegeneration: Roles of obesity, type 2 diabetes mellitus and non-alcoholic steatohepatitis. Current Opinion in Investigational Drugs. 2009;**10**:1049-1060

[2] Fabbrini E, Sullivan S, Klein S. Obesity and non-alcoholic fatty liver disease: Biochemical, metabolic, and clinical implications. Hepatology. 2010;**51**:679-689

[3] Bleich SN, Cutler D, Murray C, Adams A. Why is the developed world obese? Annual Review of Public Health. 2008;**29**:273-295

[4] Brody J. The global epidemic of childhood obesity: Poverty, urbanization, and the nutrition transition. Nutrition Bytes. 2002;**8**:1-7

[5] Roberts EA. Non-alcoholic fatty liver disease (NAFLD) in children. Frontiers in Bioscience. 2005;**10**:2306-2318

[6] Vos MB, McClain CJ. Nutrition and non-alcoholic fatty liver disease in children. Current Diabetes Reports. 2008;**8**:399-406

[7] Bellentani S, Scaglioni F, Marino M, Bedogni G. Epidemiology of non-alcoholic fatty liver disease. Digestive Diseases. 2010;**28**:155-161

[8] Younossi ZM, Koenig AB, Abdelatif D, Fazel Y, Henry L, Wymer M. Global epidemiology of non-alcoholic fatty liver disease-meta-analytic assessment of prevalence, incidence, and outcomes. Hepatology. 2016;**64**:73-84

[9] Martins IJ. Increased risk for obesity and diabetes with neurodegeneration in developing countries. Journal of Molecular and Genetic Medicine. 2013;**S1**:001

[10] Martins IJ. Unhealthy nutrigenomic diets accelerate NAFLD and adiposity in global communities. Journal of Molecular and Genetic Medicine. 2015;**9**:1-11

[11] Martins IJ. Appetite control with relevance to mitochondrial biogenesis and activation of post-prandial lipid metabolism in obesity linked diabetes. Annals of Obesity and Disorders. 2016;**1**:1-3

[12] Martins IJ. Diet and nutrition reverse type 3 diabetes and accelerated aging linked to global chronic diseases. Journal of Diabetes Research and Therapy. 2016;**2**:1-6

[13] Martins IJ. Food intake and caffeine determine amyloid beta metabolism with relevance to mitophagy in brain aging and chronic disease. European. Journal of Food Science and Technology. 2016;**4**:11-17

[14] Martins IJ. Caffeine consumption and induction of obesity in the developed world. Annals of Obesity Disorders. 2017;**2**:1-3

[15] Jensen KJ, Alpini G, Glaser S. Hepatic nervous system and neurobiology of the liver. Comprehensive Physiology. 2013;**3**:655-665

[16] Gimble JM, Sutton GM, Ptitsyn AA, Floyd ZE, Bunnell BA. Circadian rhythms in adipose tissue: An update. Current Opinion and Clinical Nutrition and Metabolic Care. 2011;**14**:554-561

[17] Buijs RM, Escobar C, Swaab DF. The circadian system and the balance of the autonomic nervous system. Handbook of Clinical Neurology. 2013;**117**:173-191

[18] Kennedy OJ, Roderick P, Poole R, Parkes J. Coffee, caffeine and non-alcoholic fatty liver disease? Therapeutic Advances in Gastroenterology. 2016;**9**:417-418

[19] Chen S, Teoh NC, Chitturi S, Farrell GC. Coffee and non-alcoholic fatty liver disease: Brewing evidence for hepatoprotection? Journal of Gastroenterology and Hepatology. 2014;**29**:435-441

[20] Patell R, Dosi R, Joshi H, Sheth S, Shah P, Sarfaraz S. Non-alcoholic fatty liver disease (NAFLD) in obesity. Journal of Clinical and Diagnostic Research. 2014;**8**:62-66

[21] Wong RJ, Ahmed A. Obesity and non-alcoholic fatty liver disease: Disparate associations among Asian populations. World Journal of Hepatology. 2014;**6**:263-273

[22] Targher G, Byrne CD. Obesity: Metabolically healthy obesity and NAFLD. Nature Reviews Gastroenterology and Hepatology. 2016;**13**:442-444

[23] Ezzat WM, Ragab S, Ismail NA, Elhosary AY, AM NEAEB, et al. Frequency of non-alcoholic fatty liver disease in overweight/obese children and adults: Clinical, sonographic picture and biochemical assessment. Journal of Genetic Engineering and Biotechnology. 2012;**10**:221-227

[24] Suano de Souza FI, Silverio Amancio OM, Saccardo Sarni RO, Sacchi Pitta T, Fernandes AP, Affonso Fonseca FL, et al. Non-alcoholic fatty liver disease in overweight children and its relationship with retinol serum levels. International Journal of Vitamin Nutrition Research. 2008;**78**:27-32

[25] Kim NH, Kim JH, Kim YJ, Yoo HJ, Kim HY, Seo JA, et al. Clinical and metabolic factors associated with development and regression of non-alcoholic fatty liver disease in non-obese subjects. Liver International. 2014;**34**:604-611

[26] Acheson KJ, Gremaud G, Meirim I, Montigon F, Krebs Y, Fay LB, et al. Metabolic effects of caffeine in humans: Lipid oxidation or futile cycling? American Journal of Clinical Nutrition. 2004;**79**:40-46

[27] Martins IJ. Caffeine consumption with relevance to type 3 diabetes and accelerated brain aging. Research and Reviews: Neuroscience. 2016;**1**:1-5

[28] Ricchi M, Odoardi MR, Carulli L, Anzivino C, Ballestri S, Pinetti A, et al. Differential effect of oleic and palmitic acid on lipid accumulation and apoptosis in cultured hepatocytes. Journal of Gastroenterology and Hepatology. 2009;**24**:830-840

[29] Gambino R, Bugianesi E, Rosso C, Mezzabotta L, Pinach S, Alemanno N, et al. Different serum free fatty acid profiles in NAFLD subjects and healthy controls after oral fat load. International Journal of Molecular Science. 2016;**17**:479

[30] Puri P, Wiest MM, Cheung O, Mirshahi F, Sargeant C, Min HK, et al. The plasma lipidomic signature of non-alcoholic steatohepatitis. Hepatology. 2009;**50**:1827-1838

[31] French MA, Sundram K, Clandinin MT. Cholesterolaemic effect of palmitic acid in relation to other dietary fatty acids. Asia Pacific Journal of Clinical Nutrition. 2002;**11**(Suppl. 7):S401-S407

[32] Clandinin MT, Cook SL, Konard SD, French MA. The effect of palmitic acid on lipoprotein cholesterol levels. International Journal of Food Science Nutrition. 2000;**51**(Suppl):S61-S71

[33] Miyoshi T, Lönnfors M, Peter Slotte J, Kato S. A detailed analysis of partial molecular volumes in DPPC/cholesterol binary bilayers. Biochimica et Biophysica Acta. 2014;**1838**:3069-3077

[34] Kheyfets BB, Mukhin SI. Simple model of local ordering of DPPC lipids in contact with cholesterol. Biochemistry (Moscow) Supplement Series A. 2015;**9**:77-83

[35] Davis CH, Berkowitz ML. Interaction between amyloid-beta (1-42) peptide and phospholipid bilayers: A molecular dynamics study. Biophysical Journal. 2009;**96**:785-797

[36] Ege C, Lee KY. Insertion of Alzheimer's A beta 40 peptide into lipid monolayers. Biophysical Journal. 2004;**87**:1732-1740

[37] Martins IJ, Fernando WMADB. High fibre diets and Alzheimer's disease. Food and Nutrition Sciences. 2014;**5**:410-424

[38] Cao C, Cirrito JR, Lin X, Wang L, Verges DK, Dickson A, et al. Caffeine suppresses amyloid-beta levels in plasma and brain of Alzheimer's disease transgenic mice. Journal of Alzheimer's Disease. 2009;**17**:681-697

[39] Arendash GW, Mori T, Cao C, Mamcarz M, Runfeldt M, Dickson A, et al. Caffeine reverses cognitive impairment and decreases brain amyloid-beta levels in aged Alzheimer's disease mice. Journal of Alzheimer's Disease. 2009;**17**:661-680

[40] Martins IJ, Lenzo NP, Redgrave TG. Phosphatidylcholine metabolism after transfer from lipid emulsions injected intravenously into rats. Implications for high density lipoprotein metabolism. Biochimica et Biophysica Acta. 1989;**1005**:217-224

[41] Dubrez L, Coll JL, Hurbin A, Solary E, Favrot MC. Caffeine sensitizes human H358 cell line to p53-mediated apoptosis by inducing mitochondrial translocation and conformational change of BAX protein. Journal of Biological Chemistry. 2001;**276**:38980-39807

[42] He Z, Ma WY, Hashimoto T, Bode AM, Yang CS, Dong Z. Induction of apoptosis by caffeine is mediated by the p53, Bax, and caspase 3 pathways. Cancer Research. 2003;**63**:4396-4401

[43] Hansen MK, Connolly TM. Nuclear receptors as drug targets in obesity, dyslipidaemia and atherosclerosis. Current Opinion in Investigational Drugs. 2008;**9**:247-255

[44] Harrison C. Neurodegenerative disorders: A neuroprotective role for sirtuin 1. Nature Reviews Drug Discovery. 2012;**11**:108

[45] Kawada T, Goto T, Hirai S, Kang MS, Uemura T, Yu R. Dietary regulation of nuclear receptors in obesity-related metabolic syndrome. Asia Pacific Journal of Clinical Nutrition. 2008;**17**:126-130

[46] Swanson HI, Wada T, Xie W, Renga B, Zampella A, Distrutti E. Role of nuclear receptors in lipid dysfunction and obesity-related diseases. Drug Metabolism & Disposition. 2013;**41**:1-11

[47] Cakir I, Perello M, Lansari O, Messier NJ, Vaslet CA, Nillni EA. Hypothalamic sirt1 regulates food intake in a rodent model system. PloS One. 2009;**4**:e8322

[48] Kitamura T, Sasaki T. Hypothalamic sirt1 and regulation of food intake. Diabetology International. 2012;**3**:109-112

[49] Wei D, Tao R, Zhang Y, White MF, Dong XC. Feedback regulation of hepatic gluconeogenesis through modulation of SHP/Nr0b2 gene expression by Sirt1 and FoxO1. American Journal of Physiology Endocrinology and Metabolism. 2011;**300**:E312-E320

[50] Li X. SIRT1 and energy metabolism. Acta Biochimica et Biophysica Sinica (Shanghai). 2013;**45**:51-60

[51] Chang HC, Guarente L. SIRT1 and other sirtuins in metabolism. Trends in Endocrinology and Metabolism. 2014;**25**:138-145

[52] Mayoral R, Osborn O, McNelis J, Johnson AM, DY O, Izquierdo CL, Chung H, et al. Adipocyte SIRT1 knockout promotes PPARγ activity, adipogenesis and insulin sensitivity in chronic-HFD and obesity. Molecular Metabolism. 2015;**4**:378-391

[53] Picard F, Kurtev M, Chung N, Topark-Ngarm A, Senawong T, Machado De Oliveira R, et al. Sirt1 promotes fat mobilization in white adipocytes by repressing PPAR-gamma. Nature. 2004;**429**:771-776

[54] Bordone L, Motta MC, Picard F, Robinson A, Jhala US, Apfeld J, et al. Sirt1 regulates insulin secretion by repressing UCP2 in pancreatic beta cells. PLoS Biology. 2006;**4**:e31

[55] Xu C, Bai B, Fan P, Cai Y, Huang B, Law IK, et al. Selective overexpression of human SIRT1 in adipose tissue enhances energy homeostasis and prevents the deterioration of insulin sensitivity with ageing in mice. American Journal of Translational Research. 2013;**5**:412-426

[56] Choi Y, Um SJ, Park T. Indole-3-carbinol directly targets SIRT1 to inhibit adipocyte differentiation. International Journal of Obesity (London). 2013;**37**:881-884

[57] Siersbaek R, Nielsen R, Mandrup SPPAR. Gamma in adipocyte differentiation and metabolism—Novel insights from genome-wide studies. FEBS Letters. 2010;**584**:3242-3249

[58] Körner A, Wabitsch M, Seidel B, Fischer-Posovszky P, Berthold A, Stumvoll M, et al. Adiponectin expression in humans is dependent on differentiation of adipocytes and down-regulated by humoral serum components of high molecular weight. Biochemical and Biophysical Research Communications. 2005;**337**:540-550

[59] Lee MJ, Wu Y, Fried SK. Adipose tissue re-modeling in pathophysiology of obesity. Current Opinion and Clinical Nutrition and Metabolic Care. 2010;**13**:371-376

[60] Qiao L, Shao J. SIRT1 regulates adiponectin gene expression through Foxo1-C/enhancer-binding protein alpha transcriptional complex. Journal of Biological Chemistry. 2006;**281**:39915-39924

[61] Qiang L, Wang H, Farmer SR. Adiponectin secretion is regulated by SIRT1 and the endoplasmic reticulum oxidoreductase Ero1-L alpha. Molecular and Cellular Biology. 2007;**27**:4698-4707

[62] Shen Z, Liang X, Rogers CQ, Rideout D, You M. Involvement of adiponectin-SIRT1-AMPK signaling in the protective action of rosiglitazone against alcoholic fatty liver in mice. American Journal of Physiology. Gastrointestinal and Liver Physiology. 2010;**298**:G364-G374

[63] Lancaster GI, Febbraio MA. Adiponectin sphings into action. Nature Medicine. 2011;**17**:37-38

[64] Samad F, Badeanlou L, Shah C, Yang G. Adipose tissue and ceramide biosynthesis in the pathogenesis of obesity. Advances in Experimental Medicine and Biology. 2011;**721**:67-86

[65] Błachnio-Zabielska AU, Pułka M, Baranowski M, Nikołajuk A, Zabielski P, Górska M, et al. Ceramide metabolism is affected by obesity and diabetes in human adipose tissue. Journal of Cellular Physiology. 2012;**227**:550-557

[66] Matsuura F, Oku H, Koseki M, Sandoval JC, Yuasa-Kawase M, Tsubakio-Yamamoto K, et al. Adiponectin accelerates reverse cholesterol transport by increasing high density lipoprotein assembly in the liver. Biochemical and Biophysical Research Communications. 2007;**358**:1091-1095

[67] Toth PP. Adiponectin and high-density lipoprotein: A metabolic association through thick and thin. European Heart Journal. 2005;**26**:1579-1581

[68] Bullen JW, Bluher S, Kelesidis T, Mantzoros CS. Regulation of adiponectin and its receptors in response to development of diet-induced obesity in mice. American Journal of Physiology: Endocrinology and Metabolism. 2007;**292**:E1079-E1086

[69] Polyzos SA, Kountouras J, Zavos C, Tsiaousi E. The role of adiponectin in the pathogenesis and treatment of non-alcoholic fatty liver disease. Diabetes Obesity and Metabolism. 2010;**12**:365-383

[70] Finelli C, Tarantino G. What is the role of adiponectin in obesity related non-alcoholic fatty liver disease? World Journal of Gastroenterology. 2013;**19**:802-812

[71] Pagano C, Soardo G, Esposito W, Fallo F, Basan L, Donnini D, et al. Plasma adiponectin is decreased in non-alcoholic fatty liver disease. European Journal of Endocrinology. 2005;**152**:113-118

[72] Oku H, Matsuura F, Koseki M, Sandoval JC, Yuasa-Kawase M, Tsubakio-Yamamoto K, et al. Adiponectin deficiency suppresses ABCA1 expression and ApoA-I synthesis in the liver. FEBS Letters. 2007;**581**:5029-5033

[73] Badman MK, Pissios P, Kennedy AR, Koukos G, Flier JS, Maratos-Flier E. Hepatic fibroblast growth factor 21 is regulated by PPARalpha and is a key mediator of hepatic lipid metabolism in ketotic states. Cell Metabolism. 2007;**5**:426-437

[74] Zhu S, Wu Y, Ye X, Ma L, Qi J, Yu D, et al. FGF21 ameliorates non-alcoholic fatty liver disease by inducing autophagy. Molecular and Cellular Biochemistry. 2016;**420**:107-119

[75] Dushay J, Chui PC, Gopalakrishnan GS, Varela-Rey M, Crawley M, Fisher FM, et al. Increased fibroblast growth factor 21 in obesity and non-alcoholic fatty liver disease. Gastroenterology. 2010;**139**:456-463

[76] Liu J, Xu Y, Hu Y, Wang G. The role of fibroblast growth factor 21 in the pathogenesis of non-alcoholic fatty liver disease and implications for therapy. Metabolism. 2015;**64**:380-390

[77] Tao C, Sifuentes A, Holland WL. Regulation of glucose and lipid homeostasis by adiponectin: Effects on hepatocytes, pancreatic β cells and adipocytes. Best Practice & Research: Clinical Endocrinology and Metabolism. 2014;**28**:43-58

[78] Pagadala M, Kasumov T, McCullough AJ, Zein NN, Kirwan JP. Role of ceramides in non-alcoholic fatty liver disease. Trends in Endocrinology and Metabolism. 2012;**23**:365-371

[79] Kasumov T, Li L, Li M, Gulshan K, Kirwan JP, Liu X, et al. Ceramide as a mediator of non-alcoholic fatty liver disease and associated atherosclerosis. PloS One 2015;**10**:e0126910

[80] Luukkonen PK, Zhou Y, Sädevirta S, Leivonen M, Arola J, Orešič M, et al. Hepatic ceramides dissociate steatosis and insulin resistance in patients with non-alcoholic fatty liver disease. Journal of Hepatology. 2016;**64**:1167-1175

[81] Yu C, Alterman M, Dobrowsky RT. Ceramide displaces cholesterol from lipid rafts and decreases the association of the cholesterol binding protein caveolin-1. Journal of Lipid Research. 2005;**46**:1678-1691

[82] Ali MR, Cheng KH, Huang J. Ceramide drives cholesterol out of the ordered lipid bilayer phase into the crystal phase in 1-palmitoyl-2-oleoyl-sn-glycero-3-phosphocholine/cholesterol/ceramide ternary mixtures. Biochemistry. 2006;**45**:12629-12638

[83] Castro BM, Silva LC, Fedorov A, de Almeida RF, Prieto M. Cholesterol-rich fluid membranes solubilize ceramide domains: Implications for the structure and dynamics of mammalian intracellular and plasma membranes. Journal of Biological Chemistry. 2009;**284**:22978-22987

[84] Martins IJ, Creegan R. Links between insulin resistance, lipoprotein metabolism and amyloidosis in Alzheimer's disease. Health. 2014;**6**:1549-1579

[85] Martins IJ. The role of clinical proteomics, lipidomics, and genomics in the diagnosis of Alzheimer's disease. Proteomes. 2016;**4**:1-19

[86] Puig KL, Floden AM, Adhikari R, Golovko MY, Combs CK. Amyloid precursor protein and proinflammatory changes are regulated in brain and adipose tissue in a murine model of high fat diet-induced obesity. PloS One. 2012;**7**:e30378

[87] Lee YH, Martin JM, Maple RL, Tharp WG, Pratley RE. Plasma amyloid-beta peptide levels correlate with adipocyte amyloid precursor protein gene expression in obese individuals. Neuroendocrinology. 2009;**90**:383-390

[88] Vanitha S, Martin JM, Dixon AE, Ades PA, Savage PD, Spaulding L, et al. Overexpression of amyloid precursor protein in adipose tissue of obese diabetic vs. obese non-diabetic individuals. Diabetes. 2007;**56**:363

[89] Lee YH, Tharp WG, Maple RL, Nair S, Permana PA, Pratley RE. Amyloid precursor protein expression is up-regulated in adipocytes in obesity. Obesity (Silver Spring). 2008;**16**:1493-1500

[90] Freeman LR, Zhang L, Dasuri K, Fernandez-Kim SO, Bruce-Keller AJ, Keller JN. Mutant amyloid precursor protein differentially alters adipose biology under obesogenic and non-obesogenic conditions. PloS One. 2012;**7**:e43193

[91] Puig KL, Floden AM, Adhikari R. Golovko. The role of adiponectin in the pathogenesis and treatment of non-alcoholic fatty liver disease. Diabetes Obesity and Metabolism. 2010;**12**:365-383

[92] Bahceci M, Gokalp D, Bahceci S, Tuzcu A, Atmaca S, Arikan S. The correlation between adiposity and adiponectin, tumor necrosis factor alpha, interleukin-6 and high sensitivity C-reactive protein levels. Is adipocyte size associated with inflammation in adults? Journal of Endocrinological Investigation. 2007;**30**:210-214

[93] Bhaktha G, Nayak BS, Mayya S, Shantaram M. Relationship of caffeine with adiponectin and blood sugar levels in subjects with and without diabetes. Journal of Clinical and Diagnostic Research. 2015;**9**:BC01-BC03

[94] Yamashita K, Yatsuya H, Muramatsu T, Toyoshina H, Murohara T, Tamakoshi K. Association of coffee consumption with serum adiponectin, leptin, inflammation and metabolic markers in Japanese workers: A cross-sectional study. Nutrition and Diabetes. 2012;**2**:e33

[95] Seidel C, Schnekenburger M, Dicato M, Diederich M. Histone deacetylase modulators provided by mother nature. Genes and Nutrition. 2012;**7**:357-367

[96] SH S, Shyu HW, Yeh YT, Chen KM, Yeh H, Su SJ. Caffeine inhibits adipogenic differentiation of primary adipose-derived stem cells and bone marrow stromal cells. Toxicology In Vitro. 2013;**27**:1830-1837

[97] Kim AR, Yoon BK, Park H, Seok JW, Choi H, JH Y, et al. Caffeine inhibits adipogenesis through modulation of mitotic clonal expansion and the AKT/GSK3 pathway in 3T3-L1 adipocytes. BMB Reports. 2016;**49**:111-115

[98] Sinha RA, Farah BL, Singh BK, Siddique MM, Li Y, Wu Y, et al. Caffeine stimulates hepatic lipid metabolism by the autophagy-lysosomal pathway in mice. Hepatology. 2014;**59**:1366-1380

[99] Horrigan LA, Kelly JP, Connor TJ. Immunomodulatory effects of caffeine: Friend or foe? Pharmacology and Therapeutics. 2006;**111**:877-892

[100] Meli R, Mattace Raso G, Calignano A. Role of innate immune response in non-alcoholic fatty liver disease: Metabolic complications and therapeutic tools. Frontiers in Immunology. 2014;**5**:177

[101] Kong S, McBurney MW, Fang D. Sirtuin 1 in immune regulation and autoimmunity. Immunology and Cell Biology. 2012;**90**:6-13

[102] Chen X, Lu Y, Zhang Z, Wang J, Yang H, et al. Intercellular interplay between Sirt1 signalling and cell metabolism in immune cell biology. Immunology. 2015;**145**:455-467

[103] Martins IJ, Tran JML, Redgrave TG. Food restriction normalizes chylomicron remnant metabolism in murine models of obesity as assessed by a novel stable isotope breath test. Journal of Nutrition. 2002;**132**:176-181

[104] Martins IJ, Redgrave TG. A 13CO2 breath test for the assessment of remnant metabolism in mice. Journal of Lipid Research. 1998;**39**:693-699

[105] Martins IJ, Sainsbury AJ, Mamo JCL, Redgrave TG. Lipid and apolipoprotein B48 transport in mesenteric lymph and the effect of hyperphagia on chylomicron clearance in insulin-deficient rats. Diabetologia. 1994;**37**:238-246

[106] Dane-Stewart CA, Watts GF, Barrett PH, Stuckey BG, Mamo JC, Martins IJ, et al. Chylomicron remnant metabolism studied with a new breath test in postmenopausal women with and without type 2 diabetes mellitus. Clinical Endocrinology. 2003;**58**:15-20

[107] Martins IJ, Redgrave TG. Obesity and post-prandial lipid metabolism. Feast or famine? The Journal of Nutritional Biochemistry. 2004;**15**:130-141

[108] Xu F, Gao ZG, Zhang J, Rivera CA, Yin J, Weng JP, et al. Lack of SIRT1 (mammalian Sirtuin 1) activity leads to liver steatosis in the SIRT1+/− mice: A role of lipid mobilization and inflammation. Endocrinology. 2010;**151**:2504-2514

[109] Purushotham A, Xu Q, Li XL. Systemic SIRT1 insufficiency results in disruption of energy homeostasis and steroid hormone metabolism upon high-fat-diet feeding. FASEB Journal. 2012;**26**:656-667

[110] Bordone L, Cohen D, Robinson A, Motta MC, Van Veen E, Czopik A, et al. SIRT1 transgenic mice show phenotypes resembling calorie restriction. Aging Cell. 2007;**6**:759-767

[111] Ideally how many grams of fat should you consume daily. Available from: http://healthyeating.sfgate.com/ideally-many-grams-fat-should-consume-daily-5501.html

[112] Martins IJ. Nutrition therapy regulates caffeine metabolism with relevance to NAFLD and induction of type 3 diabetes. Journal of Diabetes and Metabolic Disorders. 2017;**4**:19

[113] Blanchard J. Protein binding of caffeine in young and elderly males. Journal of Pharmaceutical Sciences. 1982;**71**:1415-1418

[114] Martins IJ. Unhealthy diets determine benign or toxic amyloid beta states and promote brain amyloid beta aggregation. Austin Journal of Clinical Neurology. 2015;**2**:1060-1066

[115] Sharma B, Paul S. Action of caffeine as an amyloid inhibitor in the aggregation of Aβ16-22 peptides. Journal of Physical Chemistry B. 2016;**120**:9019-9033

[116] Martins IJ. Magnesium therapy prevents senescence with the reversal of diabetes and Alzheimer's disease. Health. 2016;**8**:694-710

[117] Kynast-Gales SA, Massey LK. Effect of caffeine on circadian excretion of urinary calcium and magnesium. Journal of the American College of Nutrition. 1994;**13**:467-472

[118] Shen H, Rodriguez AC, Shiani A, Lipka S, Shahzad G, Kumar A, et al. Association between caffeine consumption and non-alcoholic fatty liver disease: A systemic review and meta-analysis. Therapeutic Advances in Gastroenterology. 2016;**9**:113-120

[119] Shen C, Dou X, Ma Y, Ma W, Li S, Song Z. Nicotinamide protects hepatocytes against palmitate-induced lipotoxicity via SIRT1-dependent autophagy induction. Nutrition Research. 2017;**40**:40-47

[120] Tong X, Zhang D, Arthurs B, Li P, Durudogan L, Gupta N, et al. Palmitate inhibits SIRT1-dependent BMAL1/CLOCK interaction and disrupts circadian gene oscillations in hepatocytes. PloS One. 2015;**10**:e0130047

[121] Chen JX, Yan SS. Role of mitochondrial amyloid-beta in Alzheimer's disease. Journal of Alzheimer's Disease. 2010;**20**(Suppl. 2):S569-S578

[122] Koczor CA, White RC, Zhao P, Zhu L, Fields E, Lewis W. p53 and mitochondrial DNA, their role in mitochondrial homeostasis and toxicity of anti-retrovirals. American Journal of Pathology. 2012;**180**:2276-2283

[123] Park J-H, Zhuang J, Li J, Hwang PM. p53 as guardian of the mitochondrial genome. FEBS Letters. 2016;**590**:924-934

[124] Safdar A, Little JP, Stokl AJ, Hettinga BP, Akhtar M, Tarnopolsky MA. Exercise increases mitochondrial PGC-1alpha content and promotes nuclear-mitochondrial

cross-talk to coordinate mitochondrial biogenesis. Journal of Biology Chemistry. 2011;**286**:10605-10617

[125] Sen N, Satija YK, Das S. PGC-1α, a key modulator of p53, promotes cell survival upon metabolic stress. Molecular Cell. 2011;**44**:621-634

[126] Aquilano K, Baldelli S, Pagliei B, Cannata SM, Rotilio G, Ciriolo MR. p53 orchestrates the PGC-1α-mediated antioxidant response upon mild redox and metabolic imbalance. Antioxidants and Redox Signalling. 2013;**18**:386-399

[127] Martins IJ. Type 3 diabetes with links to NAFLD and other chronic diseases in the Western World. International Journal of Diabetes. 2016;**1**:1-5

[128] Martins IJ. Heat shock gene Sirtuin 1 regulates post-prandial lipid metabolism with relevance to nutrition and appetite regulation in diabetes. International Journal of Diabetes and Clinical Diagnosis. 2016;**3**:20

[129] Martins IJ. Calorie sensitive anti-aging gene regulates hepatic amyloid beta clearance in diabetes and neurodegenerative diseases. EC Nutrition. 2017;**ECO. 01**:30-32

[130] Martins IJ. Heat shock gene dysregulation and inactivation of drug therapy. EC Pharmacology and Toxicology. 2017;**ECO.01**:13-15

[131] Martins IJ. Regulation of core body temperature and the immune system determines species longevity. Current Updates in Gerontology. 2017;**1**:1-6

[132] Martins IJ. Induction of NAFLD with increased risk of obesity and chronic diseases in developed countries. Open Journal of Endocrine and Metabolic Diseases. 2014;**4**:90-110

[133] Martins IJ. Nutritional diets accelerate amyloid beta metabolism and prevent the induction of chronic diseases and Alzheimer's disease. In: The Journal for Endocrinology and Metabolism, Imprint: Photon, Peer Reviewed Indexed International Journal. Photon ebooks; 2017. p. 1-48

[134] Martins IJ. Apelinergic system defects with relevance to mental disorders in diabetes. World Journal of Psychiatry and Mental Health Research. 2017;**1**:1001

[135] Martins IJ. Defective interplay between adipose tissue and immune system induces non-alcoholic fatty liver disease. Updates in Nutritional Disorders and Therapy. 2017;**1**:3.1

[136] Pénicaud L. Relationships between adipose tissues and brain: What do we learn from animal studies? Diabetes and Metabolism. 2010;**36**(Suppl. 3):S39-S44

[137] Ramachandran A, Snehalatha C, Shetty AS, Nanditha A. Trends in prevalence of diabetes in Asian countries. World Journal of Diabetes. 2012;**3**:110-117

[138] Farrell GC, Wong VW, Chitturi S. NAFLD in Asia—As common and important as in the west. Nature Reviews Gastroenterology and Hepatology. 2013;**10**:307-318

[139] Amarapurkar D, Kamani P, Patel N, Gupte P, Kumar P, Agal S, et al. Prevalence of non-alcoholic fatty liver disease: Population based study. Annals of Hepatology. 2007;**6**:161-163

[140] LaBrecque DR, Abbas Z, Anania F, Ferenci P, Khan AG, Goh KL, et al. World gastroenterology organisation global guidelines: Non-alcoholic fatty liver disease and nonalcoholic steatohepatitis. Journal of Clinical Gastroenterology. 2014;**48**:467-473

[141] Hu FB. Globalization of diabetes: The role of diet, lifestyle, and genes. Diabetes Care. 2011;**34**:1249-1257

[142] Shi X, Xue W, Liang S, Zhao J, Zhang X. Acute caffeine ingestion reduces insulin sensitivity in healthy subjects: A systematic review and meta-analysis. Nutrition Journal. 2016;**15**:103

[143] Dewar L, Heuberger R. The effect of acute caffeine intake on insulin sensitivity and glycemic control in people with diabetes. Diabetes and Metabolic Syndrome: Clinical. Research and Reviews. 2017; Available online 23 April 2017. In Press, Accepted Manuscript. https://doi.org/10.1016/j.dsx.2017.04.017

[144] Martins IJ. Bacterial lipopolysaccharides change membrane fluidity with relevance to phospholipid and amyloid beta dynamics in Alzheimer's disease. Journal of Microbiology and Biochemical Technology. 2016;**8**:322-324

[145] Martins IJ. The future of genomic medicine involves the maintenance of sirtuin 1 in global populations. International Journal of Molecular Biology. 2017;**2**:00013

[146] How Much Fat Per Day—How Many Grams of Fat Should You Eat? http://www.acaloriecounter.com/diet/how-much-fat-per-day, Accessed 06072017, Copyright © 2007 - 2017 A Calorie Counter. All Rights Reserved. Terms Of Use

[147] Martins IJ. In: Atta-ur-Rahman, editor Nutritional and Genotoxic Stress Contributes to Diabetes and Neurodegenerative Diseases such as Parkinson's and Alzheimer's Diseases. Frontiers in Clinical Drug Research-CNS and Neurological Disorders 2015 3. pp. 158-192

[148] Tahara Y, Shibata S. Circadian rhythms of liver physiology and disease: Experimental and clinical evidence. Nature Reviews. Gastroenterology & Hepatology. 2016;**13**:217-226

[149] Burke TM, Markwald RR, McHill AW, Chinoy ED, Snider JA, Bessman SC, et al. Effects of caffeine on the human circadian clock in vivo and in vitro. Science Translational Medicine. 2015;**7**:305ra146

[150] Martins IJ. Geriatric medicine and heat shock gene therapy in global populations. Current Updates in Gerontology. 2016;**1**:1-5

[151] Scorletti E, Bhatia L, McCormick KG, Clough GF, Nash K, Hodson L, et al. WELCOME Study. Effects of purified eicosapentaenoic and docosahexaenoic acids in nonalcoholic fatty liver disease: Results from the Welcome* study. Hepatology. 2014;**60**:1211-1221

[152] Alkhouri N, Dixon LJ, Feldstein AE. Lipotoxicity in non-alcoholic fatty liver disease: Not all lipids are created equal. Expert Review in Gastroenterology and Hepatology. 2009;**3**:445-451

[153] Martins IJ, Gupta V, Wilson AC, Fuller SJ, Martins RN. Interactions between Apo E and amyloid beta and their relationship to nutriproteomics and neurodegeneration. Current Proteomics. 2014;**11**:173-183

[154] Martins IJ. Over-nutrition determines LPS regulation of mycotoxin induced neurotoxicity in neurodegenerative diseases. International Journal of Molecular Science. 2015;**16**:29554-29573

[155] Tong X, Yin L. Circadian rhythms in liver physiology and liver diseases. Comparative Physiology. 2013;**3**:917-940

[156] Gnanou JV, Caszo BA, Khalil KM, Abdullah SL, Knight VF, Bidin MZ. Effects of Ramadan fasting on glucose homeostasis and adiponectin levels in healthy adult males. Journal of Diabetes and Metabolic Disorders. 2015;**14**:55

[157] Martins IJ. The global obesity epidemic is related to stroke, dementia and Alzheimer's disease. JSM Alzheimer's Disease and Related Dementia. 2014;**1**:1010

[158] Cassidy A, Skidmore P, Rimm EB, Welch A, Fairweather-Tait S, Skinner J, et al. Plasma adiponectin concentrations are associated with body composition and plant-based dietary factors in female twins. Journal of Nutrition. 2009;**139**:353-358

[159] Markaki A, Kyriazis J, Stylianou K, Fragkiadakis GA, Perakis K, Margioris AN, et al. The role of serum magnesium and calcium on the association between adiponectin levels and all-cause mortality in end-stage renal disease patients. PloS One. 2012;**7**:e52350

[160] Sierksma A, Patel H, Ouchi N, Kihara S, Funahashi T, Heine RJ, et al. Effect of moderate alcohol consumption on adiponectin, tumor necrosis factor-alpha, and insulin sensitivity. Diabetes Care. 2004;**27**:184-189

[161] Burg VK, Grimm HS, Rothhaar TL, Grösgen S, Hundsdörfer B, Haupenthal VJ, et al. Plant sterols the better cholesterol in Alzheimer's disease? A mechanistical study. Journal of Neuroscience. 2013;**33**:16072-16087

[162] Sodhi K, Puri N, Favero G, Stevens S, Meadows C, Abraham NG, et al. Fructose mediated non-alcoholic fatty liver is attenuated by HO-1-SIRT1 module in murine hepatocytes and mice fed a high fructose diet. PloS One. 2015;**10**:e0128648

[163] Rebollo A, Roglans N, Baena M, Sánchez RM, Merlos M, Alegret M, et al. Liquid fructose down-regulates Sirt1 expression and activity and impairs the oxidation of fatty acids in rat and human liver cells. Biochimica et Biophysica Acta. 2014;**1841**:514-524

[164] Martins IJ. Magnesium deficiency and induction of NAFLD and Type 3 diabetes in Australasia. Australasian Medical Journal. 2017;**10**:235-237

[165] Martins IJ. Drug therapy for obesity with anti-aging genes modification. Annals of Obesity and Disorders. 2016;**1**:1001

[166] Martins IJ. Inactivation of anti-aging genes is related to defective drug metabolism in diabetes. International Journal of Drug Discovery. 2017;**1**:3

[167] Martins IJ. Early diagnosis of neuron mitochondrial dysfunction may reverse global metabolic and neurodegenerative disease. Global Journal of Medical Research. 2016;**2**:1-8